T0269405

Let's do audit!

A practical guide to improving the quality of medical care through criterion-based audit

Andrew Weeks, Katie Lightly and **Sam Ononge**

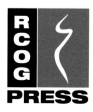

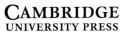

CAMBRIDGE
UNIVERSITY PRESS

University Printing House, Cambridge CB2 8BS, United Kingdom

Cambridge University Press is part of the University of Cambridge.

It furthers the University's mission by disseminating knowledge in the pursuit of education, learning and research at the highest international levels of excellence.

www.cambridge.org
Information on this title: www.cambridge.org/9781906985356

First published 2010

A catalogue record for this publication is available from the British Library

ISBN 978-1-906-98535-6 Paperback

A machine-readable catalogue record for this publication can be obtained from the British Library [www.bl.uk/catalogue/listings.html]

Published by the RCOG Press at the
Royal College of Obstetricians and Gynaecologists
27 Sussex Place, Regent's Park
London NW1 4RG

Registered Charity No. 213280

RCOG Press Editor: Jane Moody
Index: Cath Topliff MA MSocInd(Adv)
Design & typesetting: Karl Harrington, FiSH Books

Contents

Acknowledgements

We would like to thank everybody that has contributed to this book, especially Jamie Lightly, staff at Mulago National Referral Hospital, colleagues from the 'Audit in Maternity Care Project' in Uganda, Dr Sarah Blayney and everyone who helped to provide many of the examples of audit used in this book.

Introduction

This book is aimed at all those who want to improve the quality of the medical care they provide. Whether you are a nurse, doctor, manager, health-care assistant, student or laboratory technician, this book will show you how to examine the quality of the care you provide through criterion-based audit. In this process, you will decide what you should be doing in any circumstance, examine whether or not you are doing it and then look for ways of improving your care until you are doing it correctly. It has been likened to 'holding up a mirror' to your clinical practice.[1] The process is simple, free and effective. It can be carried out by anyone who wants to provide better medical care.

Although we all wish that we could provide better care it is frequently seen as someone else's problem. How often have we heard colleagues say "The care in this hospital is terrible: I wish someone would sort it out" or "If only we had the right sort of managers (or equipment, or government, or system), then our healthcare centre could be so much better"? Although it is true that leaders have a responsibility to do their best, we healthcare providers also have that responsibility. We may not have the money to buy the new expensive equipment that we want or the power to change things radically at policy level but we can all make changes in our own practice. It need not be expensive; it could be writing a guideline on a piece of paper and sticking it up on the wall, or reading up about a new development and teaching others about it, or even tying a copy of a drug formulary to the desk in the emergency room so that it is always available for staff to check the dose of prescriptions. Whatever it is, no matter how small it may seem, we can all play our part in improving practice. And we may find that a small amount of change by every healthcare professional has a far greater effect than some dramatic change by the Government – after all, there is great power in numbers. A single drop of water may seem insignificant but, when combined with many other drops, it can become a rushing river or a mighty ocean.

This book was written as the result of a training project called 'Audit in Maternity Care' which was run in Ugandan maternity units in 2001–2003.[2]

As such, many of the examples that we use relate to maternity care in African health units. The principles of audit are universal, however, and we hope that healthcare staff from every country and in every specialty will find it useful.

How to use this book

We produced the book so that it can be used either as a personal resource or as a training tool for teaching others.

The ideal way to use it is for a group to work together, each with a copy of the book. The book is divided into six lessons. Each is designed to run for about 1 hour and the group should meet together every week for 6 weeks. Before each meeting, each person in the group should read the next lesson in the book. Then, at the meeting, the group can work together through the exercises (teaching pages) which are found at the end of each lesson. You are free to photocopy these pages to hand out to the class. It is useful to discuss each question as a group in order to gain other people's opinions.

If you are working alone, read through the exercises and jot the answers down on a piece of paper before reading over the sections of the chapter where you were unsure. The answers are not provided in a block but can all be found within the text of the preceding chapter.

Managers wishing to promote audit in their organisations may decide to use this book as the basis of a 6-week course. This course does not require a teacher but will need a coordinator to monitor attendance and to produce certificates upon completion. Typically, a group would form and meet together once a week to discuss the issues and complete the exercises. It works best if the students purchase their own book at the start but the organisation agrees to refund the book cost upon successful completion of the course. This ensures that those who join are motivated and also encourages them to complete the 6 weeks.

Lesson 1.
An introduction to clinical audit

The word audit comes from the Latin word *audire* which means 'to hear'. Through the audit process, you discover or more literally 'hear' what is happening in a specific area of patient care by comparing it to accepted guidelines and standards. It is only when you know exactly what is happening in that area (and what should be happening) that you can work out what is going wrong and how you can improve it (Box 1).

Box 1. The aims of audit
■ To improve patient outcomes
■ To promote the cost effective use of resources
■ To provide education
■ To empower health care staff
■ To encourage reflection on one's own practice

It is easy to be misled into thinking that you already know why there are shortfalls in patient care. However, it is only when you have properly investigated a problem through performing an audit that you can really understand the barriers to good patient care and how to overcome them.

A formal definition of clinical audit is as follows: 'a quality improvement process that seeks to improve patient care and outcomes through systematic review of care against explicit criteria and the implementation of change'. The definition goes on to say: 'aspects of the structure, process and outcomes of care are selected and systematically evaluated against explicit criteria. Where indicated, changes are implemented to an individual, team or service level and further monitoring is used to confirm improvement in healthcare delivery'.[3]

The process of audit is typically described as an 'audit cycle' (Figure 1) and each part of the process will be described in a lesson in this book. The first

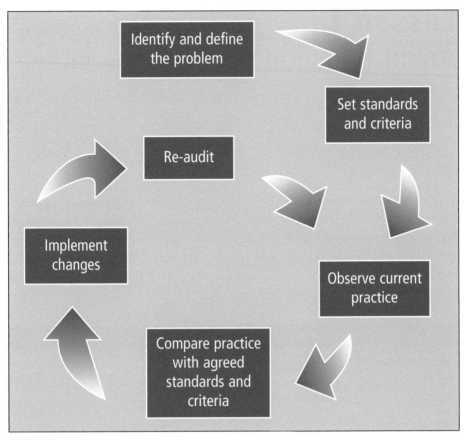

Figure 1. **The audit cycle**

step is to identify the problem to be audited (lesson 2). Standards or criteria must then be set which describe the ideal practice (lesson 3). Once these have been identified, the cycle is entered. Information is gathered about what is currently done (lesson 4) and the data are analysed and compared with the standards originally set (lesson 5). If there are any deficits, methods of improvement should be decided upon. These changes should then be implemented and the process re-audited to assess whether the changes made have led to any improvements in care (lesson 6). Ideally, the cycle should go on and on, with a continuous process of re-evaluating the situation as time goes by. Each of these steps will be discussed in greater detail in the book. In the appendix at the back of the book, a number of worked examples are provided.

Common types of clinical audit

Critical incident or adverse event audit

Critical incident or adverse event audit involves the identification of patients where an adverse (bad) event or outcome, such as severe morbidity or death, has occurred. The management of these identified cases is reviewed by a panel of healthcare professionals to identify substandard care and to learn lessons for the future management of similar cases. It helps by identifying the avoidable factors in that particular case.

The best example of a critical event audit is the Confidential Enquiry into Maternal Deaths which was introduced in the UK as early as 1952.[4] As maternal deaths are now rare in the developed world, cases of severe morbidity or 'near misses' are often audited instead.

Case notes review

The case notes review involves regular presentation of cases within units for analysis and discussion. It includes checking that all the necessary admission procedures were performed and how the current management was initiated. It often involves the presentation of rare or interesting cases – but the detailed review of a selection of regular patients is often just as revealing.

Criterion-based audit

Criterion-based audit is the most commonly used type of audit. It follows the steps of the classic audit cycle. The quality of care is assessed objectively against previously agreed criteria. The criteria are developed by a multi-disciplinary team using a systematic review of literature or evidence-based guidelines. This book focuses purely on this type of audit.

Classification of criterion-based clinical audit

Criterion-based audit can be classified into:

- **audit of structure** – examining the organisation or resources (what is available)
- **audit of process** – examining the activities themselves (what you do)
- **audit of outcome** – examining the effectiveness of activities on individuals and communities (what are the results).

Audit of structure

The term 'structure' relates to the actual facilities provided in a healthcare setting, such as buildings, theatres, staff or equipment. It may mean different things at different levels of the healthcare system. For example, at a district level you may ask whether there are enough health centres for the population while, within a hospital, you may want to know whether there are enough trained staff to run each ward or enough theatre beds to cope with the volume of work.

Audit of structure is sometimes regarded as an administrative area but it is just as important as that of process and outcome. Problems uncovered in the other audit types (process and outcome) commonly have their origin in a faulty structure.

Audit of process

Audit of process is the most frequently conducted type of clinical audit. It looks at the actual process of clinical care, examining whether there is 'good practice'. Process audits can be divided into a number of specific areas:

- **Administrative,** such as delays in appointments, waiting times, cancelled clinics
- **Notes and correspondence,** such as completion and legibility of clinical notes, whether entries are signed, dated and timed, and whether appropriate information was provided on discharge
- **Resource usage,** such as the indications for use of a test such as ultrasound or of a particular antibiotic
- **Criteria used for diagnosis,** such as making a diagnosis of a urinary tract infection
- **Management of a clinical condition,** such as postpartum haemorrhage or pre-eclampsia – are they being managed in accordance with local guidelines?

Audit of outcome

An audit of outcome examines the final impact or results of the clinical care process. The result may be seen in its effect on an individual patient, on a group or on a whole community. For example, you might audit satisfaction rates among clinic attendees, the complication rates of surgery or the number of children who have been vaccinated against measles in your community.

This is indisputably the most important area to audit but it is often the most difficult to perform. As with all audits, the outcome measures have to be set against generally accepted standards. This is sometimes called 'bench mark up'.

Do we know that audit works?

Clinical audit is a widely accepted process in Western clinical health care. Indeed, doctors in many developed countries are expected to complete audit as part of their routine duties. Clinical audit was studied extensively in the 1990s and is reviewed in a useful book called *Principles for Best Practice in Clinical Audit,* produced by the UK National Institute for Clinical Excellence.[3]

There are many examples of audit working well to improve quality. Over 100 randomised clinical trials have now been conducted examining the effectiveness of audits of practice with feedback of the results to the staff. Disappointingly, they show only a 'small to moderate benefit' from this process.[5] The review suggests, however, that the effect may be much larger when the baseline quality is low and when feedback is provided more intensively. This is supported by a large randomised trial in Argentina which has shown major benefits of a 'multifaceted approach' to behaviour change in labour ward practice.[6] The intervention included selection of opinion leaders, interactive workshops, training of manual skills, one-on-one academic visits with hospital birth attendants, reminders and feedback. The effects were dramatic: the rate of prophylactic oxytocin use increased from 2% to 84% and the episiotomy rate decreased from 41% to 30% at hospitals receiving the intervention. The rates of both remained stable at control hospitals. These effects were still seen 12 months later.

In obstetrics, high-quality care is a key requirement for reducing maternal mortality and morbidity. Critical event audit was first introduced in the UK in the 1950s.[4] This audit may have been partially responsible for the remarkable reductions in maternal mortality at this time. Since then, health care in the UK has advanced and the focus of audit has moved to improving morbidity rates, cost effectiveness and patient satisfaction.

There have been fewer audits conducted in low-resource settings, even though the evidence above suggests that this is where they may have the most effect. Indeed, there have been dramatic improvements in the quality of care demonstrated in some settings. In Uganda, the authors conducted a criterion-based audit into pre-eclampsia care and found impressive improvements in process indicators with few associated costs.[7] Similar improvements have been reported in Tanzania,[8] Mozambique[9] and Ghana.[1] The audit project in Ghana first coined the phrase 'holding up a mirror' because the very process of clearly seeing your own practice made you want to improve.

The experience of those conducting audit in low-resource settings is that, as well as being effective, the process can be both low cost and empowering for the health workers. In the Ugandan Audit in Maternity Care project, the project from which this book stems, the empowerment of health workers involved was clearly evident:

> 'Staff at all levels found that problems that they thought required large amounts of money and the work of powerful politicians to solve can often be tackled from below. Often an apparently insurmountable problem can be improved by surprisingly simple acts – a guideline posted on the labour suite wall, the repair of a broken machine, allowing women to keep their placentas after delivery as an incentive for institutional delivery, making accessible the equipment from the ward sister's cupboard and regularly checking stocks. Because these small improvements can be made cheaply and by many members of staff, the combined effect can be impressive.'[7]

Graham points out that, although sometimes substandard care is caused by the need for additional drugs and equipment, improving it is not inherently expensive in a setting where basic amenities are available.[10] Rather, it is usually caused by delays in starting appropriate care: drugs must be located or purchased or unlocked, operating rooms must be cleaned, doctors and other key staff must be found.

Who should do audit?

Everyone! Audits can range from very simple and small to massive and complicated. They can be performed by those inside an organisation or by an external group. They can be carried out by anybody: not just doctors, nurses and midwives but also students, allied health professionals, support staff and clerical workers. Anyone involved in patient care can and should be involved in the audit process.

The audit process is adaptable to all situations, as it does not give standard answers but enables those performing it to develop local solutions to local problems. It is therefore relevant to all healthcare providers within all parts of the system, from nursing and midwifery assistants to teaching hospital consultants. It is especially beneficial in rural situations where there are specific local needs which need to be assessed.

What is the difference between audit and research?

Research is the systematic and rigorous process of enquiry that aims to describe processes and develop explanatory concepts and theories to contribute to a scientific body of knowledge. Research aims to discover something new or to find out whether an untested technique actually works. Audit is about maintaining and achieving quality, through review, monitoring and evaluation against agreed standards. Put simply, research discovers what we should be doing while audit checks to see whether we are doing it. An outline of the differences between research, audit and service evaluation are shown in Table 1.

Clinical audit is not...

Blame

Every occurrence of substandard care is multifactorial, without exception. Blame is a concept that should not enter the discussion within audit. It is not useful, as it focuses all the attention on one person rather than analysing the processes and people that allowed the deficit to occur. When this happens, the system which allowed for the error will not be improved and the error is sure to repeat itself. When a serious error occurs resulting in a bad outcome, there are inevitably many people and processes involved and all could have stopped the bad outcome from occurring. But the same is true for even simple human error like prescribing the wrong medication: even simple drug errors should be preventable.

Let's examine the reasons why a patient might be given the wrong drug. One doctor may have prescribed the wrong drug and it may be tempting to simply blame this doctor. But human errors will always occur and there should have been a variety of back-up systems in place to prevent accidents occurring as a result of human error. Human error should be minimised by the doctors being alert and fresh – this is unlikely after a long weekend on call with little sleep. There should be guidelines easily available to check drug doses and senior doctors available in case of uncertainty. There should be two nurses to check the drug, both of whom should have spotted the error and alerted the doctor. The pharmacist should also check the drug. The patient also has some responsibility to ask what the drug is for and why they need it. So there should be a variety of checks in place.

Table 1. The differences between research, audit and service evaluation (derived from the UK National Research Ethics Service leaflet, *Defining Research*)[11]

Research study	Audit	Service evaluation
The attempt to obtain new knowledge. Includes studies that aim to generate hypotheses, as well as studies that aim to test them.	Designed and conducted to produce information to inform delivery of best care.	Designed and conducted solely to define or judge current care.
Quantitative research: designed to test a hypothesis. Qualitative research: identifies and explores themes following established methodology.	Designed to answer the question: 'Does this service reach a predetermined standard?'	Designed to answer the question: 'What standard does this service achieve?'
Addresses clearly defined questions, aims and objectives.	Measures against a standard.	Measures current service without reference to a standard.
Quantitative research: may involve evaluating or comparing interventions, particularly new ones. Qualitative research: usually involves studying how interventions and relationships are experienced.	Involves an intervention already in use chosen by the healthcare professional and patient.	
Usually involves collecting data that are additional to those for routine care but may include data collected routinely. May involve treatments, samples or investigations additional to routine care.	Usually involves analysis of existing data but may include administration of simple interview or questionnaire.	
Quantitative research: study design may involve allocating patients to intervention groups. Uses a clearly defined sampling framework underpinned by conceptual or theoretical justifications.	No allocation to intervention groups: the healthcare professional and patient have already chosen the intervention.	
May involve randomisation.	No randomisation.	
Usually requires ethical review.	Does not normally require ethical review.	

Human errors will always occur but a good healthcare system will have enough checks in place to prevent them leading to disaster. Even if it seems obvious that one person is to blame for a mistake, pointing the finger at them will probably not improve the situation. Another practitioner may well make the same error when put into the same situation. It is very easy to think 'I would never do that' but, if the process is flawed, it may be that you would. Audit should therefore always focus on the process rather than the individual.

Inspection from authorities

Audit should empower those working day to day to see an element of practice that could be improved and work out how best to improve it. This is most successfully performed 'in house' where local solutions to local problems can be found. External inspections decrease morale, detract attention from clinical care and make staff defensive. If they cannot be avoided, then best to make them unannounced and supportive. The best audits however come from within the local organisation.

Exercises

Exercise 1: The meaning of audit

1. Discuss the meaning of audit.

2. What is the definition of audit?

3. Look at the definition of audit on page 1 carefully and discuss the meaning of each of the following:
   - 'critically'
   - 'systematically'
   - 'own professional activities'
   - 'commitment to improving performance'
   - 'quality of care'
   - 'cost-effectiveness of care'.

4. What other types of audit have you heard of? In what ways are they the same as clinical audit?

Exercise 2: The audit diagram

1. Complete the audit diagram on the next page:

2. Discuss each box in turn:
   - What does each step mean?
   - How can each step be completed?
   - How can you organise your organisation so that a continuous cycle is set up?

3. Discuss each box in turn:
   - What problems could you have with an audit?
   - How could each step produce conflict, errors or bad feeling?
   - How can these be avoided?

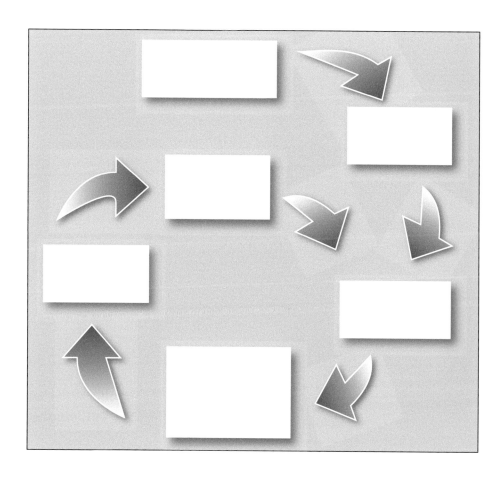

Lesson 2.
Problem identification

When you first start to do audit it can seem difficult to know where to begin. In this chapter we take you through the steps of choosing which problems to audit. As you become more experienced, it is not necessary to think at length about all of these steps: it will quickly become clear which problems should be audited and why.

Every health facility in the world can be improved – there is no such thing as a perfect healthcare system. There will be hundreds or thousands of small (or big) problems in each unit which warrant further investigation through an audit. The trick is choosing which one to start with.

Step 1 – How can we identify problems?

There are many problems which warrant audit. They could be noticed by you or by other health professionals, including students, nurses, midwives, doctors, managerial and clerical staff. They could be noted in handover meetings, ward rounds or staff meetings. Senior staff and supervisors often identify problems easily through the observation of staff and processes over a longer period of time but problems could also be noted by patients or their relatives. They could even be highlighted by the media through newspaper reports or on television. Issues could be raised by the Government as matters of national concern or through the introduction of new guidelines or national initiatives.

Issues noted by staff can easily be identified through listening carefully to discussions in meetings and ward rounds. However, feedback from clients (patients) may not be so obvious and may have to be specifically sought. The client is the most important customer; staff must find out what clients want and need and their opinions of the services being provided.

It is possible to get information from clients from informal discussion. However, formal tools such as client interviews, suggestion boxes and questionnaires can be very useful (these are discussed in lesson 4). Feedback from the community at large can also give valuable information.

Step 2 – Is the problem important enough to audit?

It can take a lot of time to carry out an audit so you have to be sure that the audit is worthy of your time. You must pick the right problem if you are going to achieve a significant impact on patient care. Common 'important' problems include:

- **serious** problems – bad outcomes, such as severe morbidity or mortality
- **common** problems in your patient group, such as pre-eclampsia or infection
- **preventable** complications that could be avoided, such as puerperal sepsis
- **recurring** problems when the same problem happens again and again (like running out of specific supplies).

Step 3 – Is further investigation warranted?

Audit is a process of investigating and understanding a problem to try to improve it. For example, complicated issues such as maternal death should always be investigated to find out exactly what happened at each stage and why, so that the same mistakes do not occur again. Other more straightforward problems do not need to be investigated to work out a solution. For example, if there is a simple problem like a spill of water on the floor – just clear it up. It will only require audit if the problem becomes recurrent or serious.

Audit can also be used as evidence to document and prove that something is happening. For example, you might have noticed that, in many instances of maternal death in a low-resource setting, the mother needed a blood transfusion which was not available. If you start a regular maternal death audit and document how many of these mothers needed blood transfusions and how many deaths were directly attributed to lack of blood transfusion, you will have evidence which cannot be ignored. This can be used to help to inform management, to liaise with other departments and to feedback to the Government to solve the problem at a higher level. If you simply say what is happening without evidence, it is easier for those in authority to ignore problems and not act on them.

Step 4 – Is it practical to audit the problem?

Simple and effective audits that yield fast results are often better than complicated elaborate audits which require a large amount of data collection. When complex audits are carried out, you may have no energy left to implement changes by the time you have finished the long process of data collection. Thus, you need to be clear from the beginning that it is feasible to carry out the audit. This is done by considering the steps involved in collecting the data at the start, before you develop the original idea too much. If you find that the original idea is too complex, either simplify the evidence that you need to obtain, concentrate on one aspect of the problem or think of a different problem to audit.

You need to be realistic when considering the practicalities. If the audit becomes very time consuming or the cases are difficult to find, it may well not be a good use of your time. For example, to investigate perceptions and experiences of women who had undergone a procedure in your healthcare facility, you could consider:

- How can you access this patient group after the procedure?
- How long do they stay on the ward after it?
- Do they attend a follow-up clinic? Where? Can you access these records?
- If not, how else can you find them? Community clinics? Baby clinics?
- Do you have the resources to find them in the community?
- Do you have any contact details for them?

If the population group attends a follow-up clinic then this audit may be feasible. However, if they do not, it would be very difficult to find these women and therefore not feasible to carry out the audit quickly and easily.

Step 5 – Can auditing improve the problem?

Although auditing often reveals aspects of care that could be improved, the solution may be out of reach of the individual facility. For example, if it is already widely known that there is no running water in a rural health facility and none in that entire area, then there is no point in auditing the problem as, at a facility level, you could not change this problem. However, if the problem is that running water is present but people do not wash their hands regularly, then it may be useful to investigate this through an audit of practice. Even the process of audit and documentation may in itself implement change, as people would be reminded of the importance of hand washing. Box 2 shows some commonly identified causes of problems in health units.

Box 2. Common causes of problems in health units	
People	Doctors, nurses, technicians (and patients); for example, the doctor not fully examining the patient; delays in initiating the treatment; unavailability of the laboratory technician/anaesthetists; the patient not seeking care promptly owing to a lack of understanding of the severity of the problem.
Machines/equipment	Can be faulty, not in good working order or not accessible; for example, monitoring equipment is kept locked in cupboards; postoperative wound sepsis may be increased because the steriliser is not maintaining the required sterilisation pressure.
Materials/supplies	Inadequate supplies may be given or distributed; for example, there may be a lack of blood in the blood bank, a shortage of long gloves for manual removal of placenta or no oxytocin available.
Methods/techniques	Different, inappropriate or outdated methods may be used for diagnosis or management; an example of this might be the use of diazepam in the management of eclamptic fits instead of magnesium sulphate.
Investigations	Measurements can be faulty, biased or inaccurate; examples of this are an inaccurate haemoglobin-measuring machine or inaccurate results from a poorly performed ultrasound scan.
Environment	There may be an incorrect ambiance, inadequate space, not enough beds or overcrowding; for example, it may be too hot or too cold for the health worker to work effectively, it may be so busy that things are omitted or the environment may be so confusing that workers cannot effectively carry out proper patient management.

Prioritising problems for audit

After identifying problems and going through the above steps, you should have already decided upon which ones require audit. If possible, a group of people should make the decision, so that several opinions are taken into account and people feel involvement and ownership of the audit. Then, as a team, the problems can be prioritised according to how manageable they will be and how important they are for quality improvement in your unit. Then you are ready for the next step of the audit cycle.

Tips for identifying problems

- Remember that process indicators are usually easier to audit than outcome indicators.
- Try to think about problems which are important and which you think can be easily improved on.
- Make your initial audits small and simple. It is far better to have a small audit which is performed well, is effective at raising standards and is completed, than to choose a grand, complicated audit that you abandon halfway through.
- When choosing a problem for a clinical audit project, it is also worth checking whether someone else locally has already started working on it.

Key points for identifying problems

- Identify possible auditable problems.
- Consider whether the problem is important enough to audit.
- Consider whether further investigation of the problem is warranted.
- Consider whether it is practical to audit the problem.
- Consider whether auditing can improve the problem.

Exercises

Exercise 3: Identifying problems

1. Consider the following problems which may occur in health units and discuss how they affect the unit in which you work:

    a. Running out of equipment or drugs.

    b. Hospital-acquired infection.

    c. Long waiting times in the outpatient department.

    d. Staff sickness.

    e. Haemorrhage (e.g. postpartum or postoperative).

2. Decide which problems from the list above you would audit and why. Which would be the most important to start with and why?

Exercise 4: Prioritisation

1. Try to think of five different problems in your own unit.

2. For each problem discuss:

    a. Is it important?

    b. Is further investigation warranted?

    c. Is it practical to audit this problem?

    d. Could auditing improve the problem?

3. Of the five problems you have identified, which two would be the best to audit and why?

These problems will be used again in future chapters so write them down and bring them to future training sessions.

Lesson 3. Setting standards and establishing criteria

Central to any clinical audit and, in particular, criterion-based audit, is knowledge and recognition of the 'standards of care' for a particular condition. Once it is established exactly what should be done, then you can compare this with what is currently done and work out how to make improvements.

There are three simple steps to this part of the audit cycle: firstly you need to find reliable, up-to-date information about the subject. Then, using this information, you can define the audit criteria. The final step is deciding how frequently you should meet the criteria for the standard of care to be acceptable.

Criteria and standards

These two words – criteria and standards – have different meanings, which also can differ between different professional groups (note that 'criteria' is the plural of 'criterion').

Audit criteria are explicit statements which define what is being measured; they represent elements of care that can be objectively measured. A criterion can be defined as a systematically developed statement that can be used to assess the appropriateness of specific healthcare decisions, services and outcomes. Criteria can also be classified into those concerned with:

- structure (what is available)
- process (what you do)
- outcome of care (what the results are).

A standard is defined as 'the level of care to be achieved for any particular criteria'. In other words, criteria are those aspects of care that you wish to examine, whereas standards are the pre-stated or implicit levels of success that you wish to achieve. For example, if you are preparing an audit of written communcations between a health centre and a hospital:

Criterion: patients referred in an emergency should carry with them a referral letter.

Standard: At least 90% of patients referred in an emergency should carry with them a referral letter.

Step 1 – Find the guidelines and evidence

Once a topic or problem has been chosen for clinical audit, valid criteria must be selected for improvement in quality of care. The criteria must be:

- based on evidence
- based on best practice
- related to important aspects of care
- capable of being measured
- acceptable to all participating staff
- realistic for the capacity of your facility.

Most of the time, existing clinical guidelines can be used to form the criteria, either directly or in a modified form. It is better to use written guidelines wherever possible, as they should be evidence based, unbiased and written and checked by experts on the subject. Many guidelines now include suggestions for audit criteria. Guidelines are often available locally within each health unit. If not, they can be obtained nationally from government departments or internationally from bodies such as the World Health Organization (WHO) or the International Federation of Obstetrics and Gynecology (FIGO).

Guidelines should be accessible to all staff, either in the library or through a manager's office. The internet also hosts many different guidelines – it is just a question of finding the right one. A good starting point is often a search engine: **www.google.com** or **www.scholar.google.com** (type in what you are looking for and then click on the correct link). An excellent list is also available in an article on searching the internet for evidence-based medicine published in *BJOG* in 2009.[12] Some commonly used sources of guidelines are given in Box 3.

You can devise criteria without using guidelines but this is time-consuming and requires considerable expertise. Ideally, those developing them should be trained in the processes of evaluating evidence from literature and grading criteria by the strength of evidence. Information from specific

Box 3. Sources of guidelines in obstetrics, gynaecology and general medicine

WEBSITES

www.cochrane.org Cochrane reviews are systematic reviews of many different areas.

www.library.nhs.uk/GUIDELINESFINDER The National Library of Guidelines is a collection of guidelines based on the guidelines produced by NICE and other UK national agencies. The main focus is on guidelines produced in the UK but, where no UK guideline is available, guidelines from other countries are included in the collection.

www.nice.org.uk The National Institute for Health and Clinical Excellence is an independent UK organisation responsible for providing national guidance on promoting good health and preventing and treating ill health. Crucial for everyday UK practice.

www.rcog.org.uk/womens-health/guidelines Evidence-based guidelines produced by the Royal College of Obstetricians and Gynaecologists in the UK.

www.rcog.org.uk/womens-health/clinical-guidance/non-rcog-guidelines A link to non-RCOG guidelines.

www.sign.ac.uk The Scottish Intercollegiate Guidelines Network (SIGN) develops evidence-based clinical practice guidelines for the National Health Service in Scotland.

www.nhshealthquality.org Completed and draft publications produced by NHS Quality Improvement Scotland (NHS QIS).

www.nlm.nih.gov The website of the National Library of Medicine and the National Institute of Health in the USA.

www.sogc.org/guidelines/index_e.asp Clinical guidelines from the Society of Obstetricians and Gynaecologists of Canada.

www.guideline.gov The USA National Guidelines Clearinghouse.

www.nhmrc.gov.au/publications/subjects/clinical.htm Australian National Health and Medical Research Council Clinical Practice Guidelines.

www.fhhs.health.wa.gov.au/inforx/clinical.html An Australian site bringing together guidelines from all over the world.

www.ranzcog.edu.au/publications/collegestatements.shtml The Royal Australian and New Zealand College of Obstetricians and Gynaecologists.

www.doh.gov.za/docs/facts-f.html South African guidelines.

www.emedicine.com A handy site for quick access to useful material.

BOOK

World Health Organization. *Managing Complications in Pregnancy and Childbirth. A Guide for Midwives and Doctors.* 2nd ed. Geneva: WHO; 2007.

journal articles or from good-quality systematic reviews can be used when there are no appropriate guidelines.

In some situations, implicit (unwritten) criteria have been used. This means that the criteria are provided by senior staff based on their own experience and knowledge. Reviewers must be careful to avoid bias and, wherever possible, formal written guidelines should be used instead.

Step 2 – Developing valid criteria

Once you have found the correct guideline or other information, you can use this and your pre-existing knowledge of the problem to work out a few key points. Include five to ten key points so the audit is focused on specific outcomes.

Each criterion should be very clear. The answers should either be easily categorised (have a yes/no answer) or be numerical, so that the audit is not ambiguous. You may also collect lots of other data from each patient, including general and background information, but it is crucial that you keep the key points clear and unambiguous. If you have too much information it is easy to get confused and forget which were the most important points.

It may also be necessary to provide a definition for elements of the criteria, so that everybody involved is clear. Remember that somebody else should be able to carry out the same audit and come up with exactly the same answers as you did.

The example in Box 4 shows how criteria were developed for an audit of the management of obstructed labour in an African health unit using WHO guidelines. The first section shows the WHO criteria for a number of conditions. Below this are the criteria that were derived from this for a unit's audit. Note how tight definitions were added to the WHO advice to provide consistency between data collectors. Note also how the criteria were adapted to the local setting where there were always long delays in obtaining a caesarean section.

Examples of criteria that should not be used include those that are:

- vague or subjective criteria, such as 'a good outcome was achieved' or 'antibiotics should be started quickly'.
- irrelevant to the acute problem, such as number of antenatal visits in a woman with a postpartum haemorrhage.
- lacking in research or agreement from experts; for example, the use of episiotomy for ventouse deliveries.

Box 4.   Criteria to include in an audit: an example for obstructed labour

The following criteria for auditing common obstetric problems are collated from various World Health Organization guidelines.

Any complication

■ Woman's history should be documented in case notes on admission (age, parity, complications in current and/or previous pregnancies).

■ General clinical state on admission should be recorded (pulse, blood pressure).

Obstetric haemorrhage

■ Intravenous access should be obtained.

■ Haematocrit or haemoglobin should be estimated.

■ Typing and crossmatching of blood should be performed.

■ Coagulation tests should be performed if indicated (clotting time, bleeding time, platelet count).

■ Crystalloids and/or colloids should be infused until crossmatched blood is available.

■ If there is continuing haemorrhage after infusion of up to three litres of fluids, blood must be given (crossmatched if possible).

■ Women should be monitored clinically to detect early deterioration at least every 15 minutes for 2 hours (pulse, blood pressure).

■ Urine output should be measured hourly.

■ Oxytocics should be used in the treatment of postpartum haemorrhage.

■ Women with antepartum haemorrhage should not have a vaginal examination unless placenta praevia has been excluded by ultrasonography or unless emergency operative delivery is immediately available.

Eclampsia

■ The treatment and prophylaxis of seizures should be managed with magnesium sulphate.

■ Respiratory rate and tendon reflexes should be monitored when magnesium sulphate is used.

■ The woman should be catheterised; a fluid balance chart should be maintained for all women.

■ Haematological and renal investigation should be performed at least once (bleeding time, clotting time, platelet count, urine albumin test).

■ Delivery should be achieved within 12 hours of first convulsion.

■ Monitoring of blood pressure and urine output should continue for at least 48 hours after delivery.

> **Box 4. Criteria to include in an audit: an example for obstructed labour (continued).**
>
> **Obstructed labour**
>
> ■ Delivery of the fetus should occur within one hour of diagnosis.
>
> ■ The urinary bladder should be drained for at least seven days postoperatively.
>
> ■ An observation chart should be maintained (urine output, pulse, blood pressure, temperature).
>
> ■ Intravenous access should be obtained before transfer to theatre.
>
> ■ Typing and crossmatching of blood should be carried out.
>
> **Following review of the WHO list, the audit team developed these final audit criteria for obstructed labour**
>
> Care of all women where the diagnosis of obstructed labour has been made should include:
>
> 1. Women should be delivered within 2 hours from admission or diagnosis.
>
> 2. The urinary bladder catheter should be inserted at the time of diagnosis (defined as within 30 minutes).
>
> 3. An observation chart should be maintained.
>
> 4. Intravenous access should be obtained and 2 litres of intravenous fluids given prior to delivery.
>
> 5. Broad-spectrum antibiotics should be given prior to surgery.
>
> 6. Typing and crossmatching of blood should be carried out before surgery.

■ impractical to assess, such as correct determination of cervical dilatation during vaginal examination.

■ optional rather than essential treatment; for example, the use of the anti-shock garment for postpartum haemorrhage.

■ an investigation or procedure which is not available in your setting; for example, instant access to magnetic resonance imaging in a rural clinic.

Step 3 – Agree on standards to be met

Having agreed on the set of criteria against which the quality of care will be measured, clinicians may want to agree on a related set of numerical standards or target percentages to be met. For example, among women who have obstructed labour, the standards for the various criteria would be:

- 100% should be delivered within 2 hours of admission.
- 80% should have a Foley catheter inserted at the time of diagnosis.
- 90% should have a broad-spectrum antibiotic started before delivery.
- 100% should have resuscitation with 2 litres of intravenous fluids before surgery.

A standard should take into consideration the capacity of the facility in terms of staff and resources. Do not set standards which cannot ever be met. It is important to distinguish between current practice and that which is aspirational. Do not set standards too low either, as you can reinforce a problem by saying that low numbers are acceptable. The potential for stimulating improvement is lost if criteria are set according to what is already practised.

Tips for setting standards and establishing criteria

- Wherever possible, base audit criteria on published guidelines.
- If no guidelines are available after thorough searching, reconsider whether it is still feasible and worth your time carrying out this particular audit.
- Ideally, use fewer than five criteria so the audit remains focused.
- Do not set audit criteria too high (never attainable) or too low (reinforcing bad practice).

Key points for setting standards and establishing criteria

1. Find the guidelines on how the condition should be managed.

2. From the guidelines produce criteria. These are the key points on which to focus the audit.

3. Decide upon appropriate numerical standards for each criterion.

Exercises

Exercise 5

1. Write a list of five guidelines that you are aware of and how and where to access them.

2. Does your unit have guidelines? How do you access them?

3. What is an audit criterion?

4. What is the difference between audit criteria and standards?

5. Consider the first audit problem in your unit from Exercise 4:
   a. Find the guidelines on how that condition or problem should be managed.
   b. From the guidelines, decide on five criteria.
   c. Decide upon appropriate numerical standards for each criterion.

6. Consider the second audit problem in your unit, from Exercise 4:
   a. Find the guidelines on how that condition or problem should be managed.
   b. From the guidelines decide on five criteria.
   c. Decide upon appropriate numerical standards for each criterion.

Lesson 4.
Measuring current practice

Having established criteria against which practice will be assessed, the next step is to observe current practice and to collect the raw audit data. To do this, you first have to work out what you actually want to know, from how many patients and how it is best to go about getting this information. It is then best to do a short pilot: collect the data on a few cases and then reassess your process to see if it works and is not too difficult or time consuming. You can then amend your plan and proceed to collect the rest of the data.

Step 1 – Work out what you need to know

There are three main sorts of data that you will need to collect: basic inform-ation, audit criteria and other relevant points.

Basic information

In most audits (but not all), basic demographic details are collected. This is done so that you can assess whether the group you are studying is represen-tative of the whole population. The basic patient identifiers are sex, age and patient identification number. These may be collected initially to enable data from various sources to be combined. It also helps if you need to go back and find the patient again to get missing data. But remember that specific identifiers (date of birth, hospital number) should be removed from the final data so that the information is made anonymous. Others pieces of back-ground data that may be appropriate are location, date and time of admission, referred or not, date, marital status, and medical information including diagnosis and severity of condition.

Remember that confidentiality is important and you need to take steps to protect these sensitive data. This may include storing data on paper in a locked office or creating passwords to protect the data if they are kept on a computer or on a portable data source (CD-ROM or Flash drive).

Audit criteria

As discussed in lesson 3, your audit criteria should be the key points that were decided to be most important for the audit.

Other relevant points

Often, there are other relevant factors which affect the audit but are not important enough to be one of the audit criteria. These points can also be included as long as they are relevant, there are not too many, they are not too difficult to access and do not make the audit too time consuming. For example, in an audit about puerperal sepsis, an audit criterion may be that all patients were prescribed and given timely and appropriate intravenous antibiotics. However, other relevant points could be exactly which antibiotics were prescribed and the quality of the documentation on drug administration.

Step 2 – Create an audit pro forma or data-collection table

When you are actually collecting the data it can be easy to lose track of where you are. This is best avoided by putting the data straight into a data–collection table or an audit pro forma. This can be done on a computer using a simple program with which you are familiar, such as Microsoft Excel or Word, or even a statistics program if it is accessible. If computer access is not possible then you can collect your data by hand, although it may take longer. A pro forma can be created by making a table that simply lists the information needed across the top and the patient audit number (assigned as you are performing the audit) down the side. Using a pro forma ensures that everyone is collecting the same data and that you do not miss key points. It also saves time, especially if you arrange the table or pro forma so that it follows the natural order in which you find the information in the file or interview; for example, name, identification number and next of kin information from the patient-identifier on the first page in the file, then parity, condition on admission and so on from the clerking, as shown in Table 2.

If there is a lot of information to collect, it may be easier to have a sheet of paper for each case. This spreads the information out, making it easier to read and helping to prevent mistakes. The information can then be copied into a computer database for analysis at a later date.

Table 2. A simple pro forma

Audit no.	Hospital ID no.	Sex	Parity
1			
2			
3			

Step 3 – Work out how many cases you need

Sometimes you should aim to audit all cases; for example, all cases of puerperal sepsis in the department in one week or all maternal deaths. In general, you should aim to get 25–50. If the problem is not so common, cases can be obtained over a longer period of time. In other situations where the condition is extremely common (such as perinatal deaths in large hospitals in developing countries) you can pick a representative sample instead of auditing the whole group. This means that you select a small sample from the total population and use the result from that one as an approximation. It must be chosen in a non-biased manner, such as picking every fifth one from the delivery register. The group that you pick must also be a similar population to the overall population group. The accuracy of the result from this representative sample can be improved by increasing the size of the sample and ensuring that it is randomly selected.

Formal sample size calculations can be conducted for audits but are not very useful. These calculations are beyond the scope of this book but they are described in detail by Mayo and Harvey.[13]

Step 4 – Work out the best way to find out the information

It is possible to assess current practice retrospectively or prospectively. Retrospective collection is done by looking back at data that have already been collected in the past. Prospective collection is done by assessing events as they happen, recording the data as you go along.

Retrospective collection

Retrospective collection of information can be performed by:

■ reviewing the patient's case notes
■ reviewing routinely collected data.

You can review the case notes of a patient with a particular problem; for instance, the case notes of all women who had obstructed labour in the last 6 months. You can also review the routinely collected data; for example, the data in the delivery register, admission book or hospital computer database.

The problem with retrospective data collection is that records are often inadequate and lacking the information you need. In clinical audit, all the information or activities not documented are taken as not having been performed. This may not, of course, be true but you cannot simply assume that something has been done when there is no record. It does mean, though, that you are auditing both practice and documentation. Poor documentation therefore makes it impossible to retrospectively assess the quality of practice. Through auditing, however, the standard of record keeping tends to improve.

The other problem with retrospective data collection is that of missing records. It can be difficult to find the records so, if you are looking for case notes, be sure to record all patient identifiers carefully, especially name, age, location and patient identification number. This means that the people working in the records office have as much information as possible to find the file. It is crucial to try and locate missing records. This is because missing records are often the most unusual or complicated cases and they may have been kept to one side for discussion or review. This means that many of your positive results may be lost in those missing case notes. To get data from only those notes that are easily found may give a misleading picture.

Prospective collection

Prospective data can be collected through:

■ prospective audit forms
■ interview
■ questionnaires
■ observation.

Prospective audit forms are data collection forms which are filled in as the patient uses the service. The form will usually be attached to the patient's case notes at the time of first contact and kept with them until discharge. This allows the form to be filled at the time of care, detailing, for example, times (such as arrival, first interview and treatment) or events (such as contact with staff, loss of signal on a cardiac monitor or the times when the patient is in pain). This kind of audit allows you to collect data that would not normally be collected or to use strict definitions to increase the accuracy of the data.

Interviews with staff are also a helpful way of collecting data but may also be inaccurate. Staff members may present an inaccurate impression of their performance, making it sound better or worse than it is.

Questionnaires are less time consuming than interviews as they can be sent out to many people at once. For example, a questionnaire survey of clinicians can be performed, asking them to describe aspects of their own practice. However, these often have a poor response rate of 50% or lower, with the keenest and best being over represented in the responders. Once again this distorts the results.

Observation is another way of collecting data prospectively. Watching staff at work is an indispensable source of information about their actual performance. The observation can be of the way procedures are performed, the way the care is delivered or of the clinic environment and layout. Obtaining permission from staff members and discussing the clinical audit process before the observation takes place can help to reduce anxiety. A common limitation is that some staff members feel anxious or threatened when they are observed and so do not perform in their usual way. The way to overcome this is to inform staff that observations will be taking place in a certain area in the future (at an unspecified time) but not when and not what. The person doing the observation usually does so secretly so as to gain an accurate observation of normal practice. An example of observation is the counting of operation swabs preoperatively and at closure of abdomen at caesarean section. This can be carried out by medical students. Confidentiality and anonymity are crucial here. If this is not achieved then staff may become angry and may prevent future audits.

Other sources of information

It is also important to consider the views and opinions of the users of the health service. Here are some ways of getting this information from patients and their carers:

Client interviews

Short lists of simple questions will suffice to find out what the client thinks of the quality of services. First, explain to the client why you want to do the interview and what it will entail. Also explain that what they say will be anonymous and will not affect the care that they receive in any way. Ask permission then conduct an interview using open-ended questions that will not bias the response. For example:

- What did you like about the clinic?
- What did you not like about the clinic?
- What did you expect that you did not receive?
- What have you heard about this clinic?
- What changes do you think could/should be made in the clinic?

When using client interviews, be aware of courtesy bias. Clients may not want to offend the providers and so may not give all of the negative information freely if not asked in the appropriate manner. It is also important not to take up too much of the client's time.

Focus groups

You can also get client feedback from a focus group discussion. In this, several people are brought together as a group and discussion is facilitated using a questionnaire. This method helps reduce courtesy bias and may improve recollection. Ideally, focus groups are interviewed at convenient times; for example, patients awaiting discharge from hospital or mothers waiting to have their babies immunised at mother and baby clinics.

Suggestion boxes

Some clinics have suggestion boxes that clients can use to comment anonymously on the quality of services. These must be user friendly: paper and pencils must be available and a box should be in an accessible place where staff will not know which client is making suggestions or criticising services. Staff must also make regular efforts to review the contents of the box, with a view to including clients' information in the quality improvement action plans.

A drawback of the suggestion box method is that it is not possible to discuss the suggestions or criticisms with the individuals where you need clarification. It also selects those patients who are confident to express themselves on paper and so may miss the views of others.

Community feedback

It is useful to obtain certain information from the community at large. This may include: what are their health problems, why they do or do not use health services nearest to them, what they need from the facility or what suggestions they might have for improving services.

Meetings at which the health facility representative simply asks community members for their needs and suggestions can also be useful.

Supervisors' observations

Supervision is the process of guiding, helping and teaching healthcare providers at their workplace how to perform better. Through supervision, the supervisor may be able to identify problems that may have the greatest impact upon the quality of health services.

Step 5 – Test your audit pro forma

After going through the above steps, you are ready to start interviewing or reviewing files to get the data. When you start doing this, you may find that the pro forma or the method has flaws or could be more efficient in some way. It is therefore recommended that you try out the pro forma on a few cases (about three to five) to see how it works. Review the above steps again now that you have the experience of having looked at a few cases of the audit and make any amendments to the pro forma. Then try it out again and add any details that were missed from the first few cases.

Step 6 – Collect the data

Now is the time-consuming part: collecting the data. Try to set aside a time and a quiet place where you will not be disturbed so that you can get through it as fast as possible. This part can be boring but try to look at it as a learning experience: you can compare the methods of different clinicians or try to think what you would have done. In very large or important audits, the data collection is often performed independently by two or more separate people to reduce the number of errors (double data entry). Each person will separately collect the data and then the two sets of results are compared. Where there are any differences, the original data source can be examined and the correct answer identified. This reduces mistakes due to human error.

Tips for measuring current practice

■ Set aside a time and place where you will not be disturbed, so you can gather the data as quickly as possible.
■ Be sure to arrange the pro forma in the order that you find the information in the file or the natural order of the interview. This will make it quicker to fill in.
■ Get help from colleagues if you can. This can turn a very boring process into a useful group learning session.

Key points for measuring current practice

1. Work out what you need to know:

    ■ basic data
    ■ audit criteria
    ■ other relevant points.

2. Create an audit pro forma.

3. Work out how many cases you need.

4. Work out the best way to find out the information.

5. Test the audit pro forma.

6. Collect the data.

Exercises

Exercise 6: The pro forma

1. What is an audit pro forma? Why is it useful?

2. What does retrospective data collection mean? List two examples.

3. What does prospective data collection mean? List two ways in which this might be done.

4. Consider the first audit problem in your unit from Exercise 4:
   a. List the data that you would like to collect.
   b. Create an audit pro forma.
   c. How would you find this information?

5. Consider the second audit problem in your unit from Exercise 4:
   a. List the data that you would like to collect.
   b. Create an audit pro forma.
   c. How would you find this information?

Lesson 5.
Analysing the data and comparing practice with agreed criteria

Once you have collected the information, the 'raw data', on your audit pro forma, you need to bring all the data together and organise it. Then, use some simple mathematics such as averages, percentages and totals to summarise it so that it can be easily understood and used. You can then compare this with the audit criteria and standards that you created previously (see lesson 3).

Step 1 – Gather and organise the data

First, make sure that you have all of the pieces of paper and computer files that contain the raw data. If you are missing any parts of the data, try to find them now or it can confuse you later during your analysis. If access to a computer is available, then the data can be put into a table so they are clear and the information is easy to manipulate. This is especially important when there are large patient numbers. Whether you are putting the information into the computer or not, be sure to number your cases with your own audit number, so you can easily identify each patient. For example, if you have 25 cases, number the paper or the first column of the table 1–25 in ascending numerical order and then you can remove the personal identifying information such as hospital number and date of birth from the case.

Step 2 – Work out some simple calculations

Raw data need to be summarised using simple mathematics so that they are easy to read and easy to understand, and so that patterns become easy to recognise. The most commonly used calculations are to work out averages of the figures, percentages or totals/sum. Once the calculations have been performed, the data can then easily be presented in the form of graphs and tables.

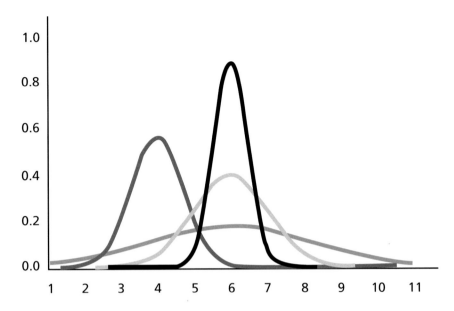

A. Examples of 'normal' distributions

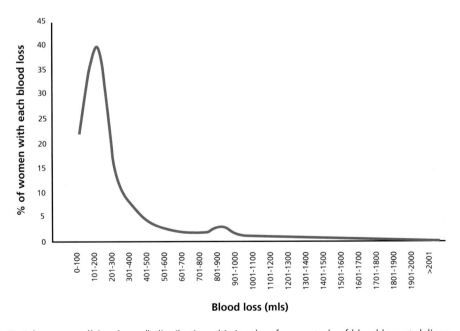

B. A 'non-normal' (or skewed) distribution; this is taken from a study of blood loss at delivery

Figure 2. **Histograms showing examples of 'normal' and 'non-normal' distribution**

Which analysis should be used for which data?

Basic demographics

Some of the data do not need to be analysed, such as the patient's number, as they are simply collected to locate the cases. The rest of the basic data should be summarised by whatever calculations are the most appropriate according to the data; for example, averages, percentages and totals.

Audit criteria

It is important to use the same calculation for the data as the audit criteria so they can be directly compared; commonly, this will be percentage versus percentage.

Other relevant points

Analyse other relevant points as for basic demographics. Some of this information can also be presented as tables or text if appropriate.

Types of data

Data can be described as continuous or categorical.

Continuous data are data for which each item is represented as a number. Examples of these data are age, pulse or time taken to treat a patient. These data can be further classified according to their distribution in the population as **'normal'** or **'non–normal'** (also known as 'skewed'). The distinction between normal and non–normal data distributions is important when it comes to the analysis of the data. There are ways of formally testing for normality but the easiest way is to see whether the most common value of the set of values is about half-way between the largest and smallest value. An alternative is to draw a histogram and look to see if it is symmetrical (Figure 2A) or not (Figure 2B). Examples of data that are usually normally distributed are age, pulse and weight. These data are best summarised using the mean value (see below).

Other continuous data sets are **'non–normal'** or **'skewed'**. This typically occurs when there is a clear cut-off at one end of the range of values and the most common value is near that end. Blood loss at delivery is a classic example. The most common value may be 200 ml but it is obviously never less than zero and may be as high as 4000 ml. Thus, the data set in the histogram is not symmetrical. These type of data are best summarised using the median value (see page 40).

Categorical data are data where every value is expressed as either 'yes' or 'no'. Thus, there are only two options for each piece of data. Examples of this are: 'age over 50?', 'satisfied?' and 'was there a good response to treatment?'. Of course, some of these need to be very carefully defined so that it is absolutely clear to everyone whether the answer for any individual is 'yes' or 'no'. However, classifying data in this way makes the analysis easy, as they can be described as a percentage for whom the answer was 'yes' (or 'no'). It also allows easy comparison with standards, as those are also usually expressed in this way.

Data can be easily switched from continuous to categorical by predefining a cut-off value. This splits the data into two groups and is a useful technique in criterion-based audit, as the standards are usually expressed in categorical terms. For example, the waiting time in an emergency department is a continuous variable. The standard may, however, be that 'not more than 10% of patients should wait for more than 4 hours'. The values for each patient will need to be reclassified according to whether their wait was over or under 4 hours. In collecting the data you may wish to collect the actual times and then categorise them later during the analysis stage of the audit. Having the data in both forms will allow you to describe the data in both continuous terms (for example, the mean waiting time was 38 minutes) and categorical terms (for instance, 29% waited over 1 hour and 8% waited over 4 hours).

More information about data descriptions and analysis can be found in standard statistical textbooks.

Summarising the data

An **average** is a value that is taken to be representative of a data set; it is a measure of the 'middle'. It is a single value that is meant to typify a list of values. The three most relevant forms of averages are referred to as measures of central location: mean, mode and median. The word 'average' is often used in place of 'mean', even though they are strictly not identical.

The **mean** is the arithmetic average of a set of values. It is the sum of the observations divided by the number of observations. The mean is calculated by adding together all of the results for one particular outcome and then dividing this by the total number of patients.

The **mode** is the value that occurs with the highest frequency in a set of values.

The **median** is the number which separates the higher half of a sample from the lower half. It can be found by arranging the values in order from the lowest value to the highest value and picking the middle one.

A worked example

An audit was performed of all of the maternal deaths in a small regional African hospital over 6 months. The audit group was looking at the data and organising them in preparation for presenting the results to the department. Table 3 gives the basic demographics of the patients.

Table 3. Audit of maternal deaths; demographics of patients

Audit no.	Name	Patient ID	Age	Parity	Referred
1	NM	2894	22	4	Y
2	PT	9362	25	1	Y
3	FM	7826	19	1	N
4	RD	3850	22	2	N
5	EM	1362	21	1	N

Here is how the group decided to summarise and analyse the data, in preparation for the presentation:

1. Audit number – this does not need to be analysed other than to get the total number of patients in the audit.

2. Name/patient identification number – again this does not need to be analysed, as the information is only used to identify patients. It was deleted from the database so that the information is anonymous.

3. Age – the different forms of average can be used. However, the fact that the median and average are the same suggests that these data are normally distributed.

    Mean: sum of ages divided by total number of patients.
    Sum of ages = 22 + 25 + 19 + 22 + 21 = 109
    Total number of patients = 5
    109 ÷ 5 = **21.8**

    Mode: each number occurs only once except 22, which occurs twice, so 22 is the most commonly occurring number and is therefore the mode.

Median: arrange the numbers into ascending numerical order and then see which one is in the middle: 19, 21, 22, 22, 25 – 22 is in the middle – the median.

4. Parity: the different forms of average can be used. However, the mean is nearly twice the value of the median value, suggesting that this dataset is not normal, it is skewed.

Mean: sum of parities divided by total number of patients.
Sum of parities = 4 + 1 + 1 + 2 + 1 = 9
Total number of patients = 5
9 ÷ 5 = **1.8**

Mode: P1 occurs 3 times, P2 occurs once and P3 occurs once, so P1 is the most commonly occurring number and is therefore the mode.

Median: arrange the numbers into ascending numerical order and then see which one is in the middle: 1, 1, 1, 2, 3 – P1 is in the middle or median.

5. Referred: these data are categorical so percentage is used.

Total number referred divided by total number of patients multiplied by 100%
Total number referred = 2
Total number of patients = 5
2 ÷ 5 = 0.4
0.4 × 100 = 40%

The group therefore summarised their data as:

■ Total number of patients = 5
■ Name/identification number – not presented
■ Mean age – 21.8
■ Median parity – 1
■ Referred – 40% were referred.

Representation of data

It is often useful to summarise the data that you have analysed through making summary tables of key points. Graphs can also be helpful, as they show the data in a more interesting and easy to read format. Key data points and graphs will be undoubtedly useful when you come to present your data to your colleagues. Preparing summary tables and graphs also helps you to understand and analyse the results better, as patterns can become more apparent.

Step 3 – Compare the results to the audit standards and identify performance gaps

Following measurement of current practice, the findings must be summarised so as to identify aspects of care which are satisfactory (better than the agreed criteria or standard) and those for which changes are required. By doing this, you are able to define the performance gap, which is the difference between the agreed standard and the current practice. The performance gaps should be expressed preferably in percentages or proportions. For example, in management of obstructed labour, the agreed standard in one audit was that the delivery of the baby within 2 hours should be achieved 100% of the time. However, if the audit found that only 40% of the babies were delivered within 2 hours, the performance gap would be 60% (100% – 40%).

In the beginning of any clinical audit cycle, the audit of current practice often gives a negative picture of the performance. After all, this is probably why you decided to audit it in the first place. So do not be discouraged, as the next measurement of current practice may show marked improvement. The key is to look critically at what is causing the performance gap and what action you can take to reduce the gap.

Tips for analysing the data and comparing practice with agreed criteria

■ Ensure that you collect all the data and organise them carefully before you start analysing them. When parts are missing this can distort the calculations and you may have to repeat them.
■ The vast majority of the calculations are very simple, consisting mostly of averages and percentages. A computer can often help you to perform these calculations, improving accuracy and saving time.

Key points for analysing the data and comparing practice with agreed criteria

1. Gather and organise the data.

2. Work out some simple calculations, then summarise the key data points in either tables or graphs.

3. Compare the results with the audit standards and identify performance gaps.

Exercises

Exercise 7: Calculations

1. What are the definitions of these calculations and how do you calculate them?

   a. Mean?

   b. Mode?

   c. Median?

   d. Percentage?

2. Consider the first audit problem in your unit from Exercise 4:

   a. Which calculations will you have to work out for each item on the audit pro forma?

   b. Why have you chosen that particular calculation?

   c. What is the best way to present these data for each item?

3. Consider the second audit problem in your unit from Exercise 4:

   a. Which calculations will you have to work out for each item on the audit pro forma?

   b. Why have you chosen that particular calculation?

   c. What is the best way to present these data for each item?

Exercises

Exercise 8: Analysis

An audit was performed of the initial management of postpartum haemorrhage over a one-week period in a regional referral hospital. The data have already been collected and the auditors are in the process of analysing them.

The audit criteria were:

i.   The team should be mobilised within 10 minutes of arrival in 100% of cases.
ii. Vital signs, especially blood pressure (BP) and pulse, should be checked within 10 minutes of arrival in 100% of cases.
iii. Intravenous (IV) access should be obtained within 10 minutes in 95% of cases.
iv. intravenous fluids should be started within 20 minutes in 80% of cases.

Audit no.	1	2	3	4	5	6	7	8
Age	21	25	28	14	17	19	32	19
Parity	1	5	6	0	1	1	6	2
Team mobilised within 10 minutes	Y	N	Y	Y	N	N	N	Y
Vital signs immediately checked	Y	N	N	N	Y	Y	Y	Y
Uterine massage	Y	Y	Y	Y	Y	Y	Y	Y
Oxytocin given	Y	Y	Y	Y	Y	N	Y	Y
IV access obtained	Y	Y	Y	N	N	N	Y	Y
IV fluids started	N	Y	Y	N	N	N	N	Y
Catheterise	Y	Y	Y	N	N	N	N	N

1. What were the mean, median and mode ages of the group?

2. What were the mean, median and mode parities of the group?

3. What percentage had vital signs checked within 10 minutes?

4. What is the performance gap for mobilising the team immediately?

5. What is the performance gap for starting of IV fluids?

The answers can be found overleaf.

Answers to Exercise 8

1. Mean = 21.9
    Median = 20 (if there are two middle values, the median is halfway between the two)
    Mode = 19

2. Mean = 2.75
    Median = 1.5
    Mode = 1

3. 5 of 8
    $5 \div 8 = 0.625$
    $\times\ 100 =$
    62.5%

4. 4 of 8
    $4 \div 8 = 0.5$
    $\times\ 100 =$
    50%
    Should be 1005; therefore performance gap is $100 - 50 = 50\%$

5. 3 of 8
    $3 \div 8 = 0.375$
    $\times\ 100 =$
    37.5%
    Should be 80%; therefore performance gap is $80 - 37.5 = 42.5\%$

Lesson 6.
Implement change and re-audit

Introduction

After all the work collecting the data for the audit is completed, it may feel as if the work is nearly over. In fact, it is only just beginning. The implementation of change is the **most important step** in the audit cycle. It is also the hardest but most rewarding step to achieve. Many factors must be considered to perform it properly. Do not forget that the reason that audit is performed is to find out what shortcomings there are in the system so that we can try to improve them. Only when it has been established exactly what suboptimal care has occurred, can we address the specific issues that have caused it and implement changes in practice.

Assuming that audit reveals some aspects of care which measure up poorly against the agreed criteria, the next step is to promote appropriate change in practice. There are five principal explanations for care falling short of agreed standards:

1. The agreed criteria are invalid or the standard is unrealistic.

2. The organisation is deficient. This could be in staff, supplies, distribution, workload or leadership.

3. Knowledge is inadequate.

4. Skills are inadequate owing to a lack of training or supervision.

5. Attitudes are inappropriate – there may be a lack of accountability, poor motivation, unmet personal needs or unclear job descriptions.

In choosing approaches that might persuade colleagues to change, it is important first to determine the reason for each deficiency. Sometimes the explanation may be glaringly obvious. More often it can be very difficult to tease out the underlying reasons. This is where the 'root cause analysis' comes in. This analysis seeks to find out the real underlying causes of the problems and the barriers to change. This will help us to design interventions to promote change.

Step 1 – Find the root cause of poor performance

Root cause analysis is the main diagnostic step in the performance improvement process. It is the transition from description of the problems to development of the solutions. Performance problems need to be attacked at their root or else they will persist.

In looking for the root cause of performance gap, an aspect of the performance improvement toolkit is useful in trying to define the root causes of the problem.[14] This method is called the 'why? why?' technique or the 'five whys' approach. It is an easy-to-use quality management technique that may be used to structure a discussion of the problems. It consists of simply asking 'why?' repeatedly until the underlying cause of a problem becomes clear. The technique encourages careful inquiry into the causes and discourages jumping to conclusions.

Those participating in the audit process and other stakeholders (see **Glossary of terms**, page 91) should meet together to identify chains of causes of the performance gap. When those can think of no more causes in one chain and no more answers to the question why, then the leader asks if there are any other causes of the gap and begins another chain (Figure 3). For example, a group in Uganda wondered why they had found long delays in starting operations. Group discussions with theatre staff, surgeons and nurses revealed the initial problems shown in Figure 4.

A root cause analysis using the 'why? why?' technique forces the quality improvement teams to consider the complexity of a problem and to take an objective look at all the contributing factors. It also helps team members to choose one or more aspects of the problem that they have some control over changing and identify those that they believe can significantly improve the situation. The purpose of audit is to bring about improvement and this step must be tackled if the exercise is not to have been a waste of valuable time.

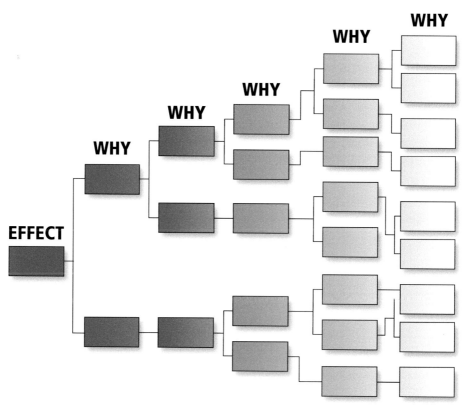

Figure 3. **The 'why? why' tree or 'five whys' approach**

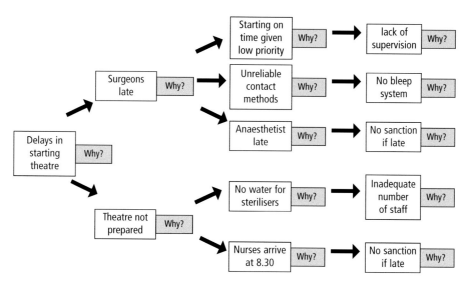

Figure 4. **Using the 'why? why' tree to reveal problems**

Step 2 – Select appropriate interventions

Having defined the root causes of the performance problems, stakeholders should use the same care in selecting interventions. The leader of the audit team encourages staff members whose performance is being analysed to suggest solutions. The people whose work has been audited have the best knowledge of their job and generally contribute the most practical ideas. Furthermore, if staff members themselves play an important role in developing solutions, they are less likely to feel that the solutions were imposed and more likely to embrace change.

In prioritising the solutions, the stakeholders should be able to answer the following questions:

- Is the proposed solution feasible?
- Will the proposed solutions actually solve the problems?
- Will the proposed solutions provide the best results for the least resources?
- Is the proposed solution acceptable to the patients, community and staff members who will carry out the solution?
- Is the proposed solution sustainable?

An example is seen in Box 5. A problem was identified that women were waiting a long time to be seen at a Ugandan antenatal clinic. After going through the 'why, why' analysis the changes identified in Box 5 were suggested and individuals were identified who had the power to implement them. While some changes could be made by the nurse in charge of antenatal clinic or junior doctors, others needed massive changes to be implemented by the Ministry of Health or even the country's President.

Looking at the suggested changes in Box 5, the ones ticked can be implemented without much difficulty. It is crucial to be realistic and practical when deciding on which interventions are the most appropriate. The ticked items can be easily carried out by staff in the hospital if they are willing but there is only a limited amount that could be done about the remaining two items marked with crosses. Do not be discouraged, though: you can still take small achievable steps to try to generate change, such as a letter to the Ministry of Health or to the media. The Government and policy makers cannot improve on problems if they do not realise what problems exist and the extent of them.

Box 5. Delays in antenatal clinic		
Change needed	**Responsible person**	
Checking that all doctors are present	Antenatal clinic manager	✓
Revising the patient visit strategy in line with new WHO policy	Consultant obstetrician	✓
Putting the guideline up on the wall	SHO in obstetrics	✓
Triple nurse numbers	The Government	✗
Shorten morning hand-over meeting	Head of department	✓
Increase funding for maternity care	President or Prime Minister	✗

Step 3 – Create an action plan

After suggesting the changes, it is advisable to identify a specific person by name to carry out a task and to give a specific timeframe in which to have completed it. This is best done in the format of an action plan.

An action plan is a simple table created by the implementation team which records clearly the problems and the plans to rectify them. It is a valuable tool for planning, implementing and monitoring activities. The elements of an action plan include:

- identification of the problem and its cause (this can be omitted if necessary)
- recommended solutions and interventions identified from the root cause analysis
- the names and contact points of the people responsible for carrying out the activities
- the deadline when the activity should be accomplished (usually the next meeting of the audit group).

An example of an action plan is illustrated in Table 4. In this situation, women who had delivered at home were arriving with postpartum haemorrhage at a remote African hospital. The problem was that there were considerable delays after reaching the hospital before they received treatment. A 'why? why?' analysis had identified a number of root causes: delays were occurring because the patients and attendants were getting lost trying to find the delivery suite, there were problems in finding their old notes (they were not allowed in before the old notes were found) and in contacting the doctors. Achievable, low-costs solutions were identified for each of these problems and an action plan drawn up (Table 4).

Table 4. Postpartum haemorrhage action plan

Problem and cause	Recommended actions	By whom	By when
Clients have problem locating services because of lack of signage	Prepare and affix signs	Mr Ssenfuka (maintenance)	30 October
Long delay at reception because of difficulty in finding client records	Remove and store (archive) obsolete records	Mr Kaggwa (medical records)	30 November
Difficulty in contacting doctor in emergency	On-call doctor will write their location on the blackboard	Mrs Kadama (labour ward sister)	26 September
	Emergency bell		

The process of producing an action plan in this format provides a clear definition of problems and solutions. It means that the appropriate course of action and priority areas are decided upon jointly and publicly by the team. A named individual should be responsible for leading or coordinating each of the actions. This makes people accountable and responsible for trying to improve the situation and ensures that it is done in a timely fashion. Remember to be realistic when deciding upon timeframes for the actions. Some steps can be taken immediately but mid-term and long-term improvements can take months or years. When it is anticipated that a goal may take a long time to achieve, it is often useful to break it down into smaller steps, each with a shorter timeframe, to ensure that the implementation stays on track. When actions are clearly defined as steps, it is far easier to carry them out and to assess whether the targets have been reached.

The next step is to complete the interventions decided upon in the action plan. It is important to keep reviewing the action plan to ensure that people are taking the actions that they are supposed to take.

Steps for effective implementation

Inform seniors and policy makers in the department

It is very difficult to change practice if the senior staff in the department are not on board. It is crucial to make sure that these senior staff are aware and involved in the audit process as much as possible. The leaders are the ones that people will listen to regarding possible change. They are also more likely to have access to any finance that may be necessary.

Raise awareness

Tell people what you are doing and why you are doing it. This simple step is free and gets people thinking about the problems. The more that people are aware of what you are doing, the more interested that they will be in your findings and in making any changes necessary. Simply getting people thinking about issues may help them to re-evaluate their own practice and perhaps improve it.

Keep data collection limited

Remember why you are performing the audit. It is easy to get carried away with data collection and not leave enough time and energy for sensitising people and implementing change. Collect enough information to prove your point and then go about trying to change things.

Present the findings

Ensure that you make a presentation of your findings to your colleagues; this can be at a specific audit meeting, a handover meeting or really any time when there is a group of staff together. The more people that hear your findings the better and the more likely that people will try to implement change. Consider different media for informing people: presentations, posters, websites, or journals. These can be local, national or international as appropriate.

Inform management of the hospital, other departments and officials

Changing some of the issues raised may be outside the remit of the auditor; government ministers, policy-makers and hospital managers may be better placed to effect change. It is therefore important to make sure that these people are aware of problems and possible ways of tackling and resolving them. Inform them by whichever method seems most appropriate: by word of mouth from the auditors or seniors, letter, email or in meetings.

Avoid blame

Remember that we all make mistakes and no one is perfect. If there have been errors then it is likely that anyone could have made them. If there was an error, do not mention the person's name. Look to ways of improving the system to prevent those errors occurring again – maybe extra teaching, guidelines, reminder charts or a system of crosschecking actions with others. All of these can prevent mistakes.

Teach

When you present your findings, ensure that you teach people about the guidelines as part of the presentation. This will increase everyone's knowledge about what should be done.

Equipment

Fix it! Where non-functioning equipment is found, endeavour to get it fixed. Liaise with the engineering or maintenance department. These steps often have significant, sustainable effects.

Meet monthly

Gather a committed group of people together and meet monthly at a time when you can all attend: maybe have a short meeting just after the morning meeting once a month so that everyone can attend or allocate an afternoon when you can have a longer meeting with presentations and discussions. Remember not to criticise people though, or they will 'vote with their feet' and find reasons not to attend.

Remind

Do not be afraid to keep asking people about their work towards the audit and whether they have achieved the tasks allocated to them in the action plan. Staff may be busy and may forget unless gently reminded.

Re-audit

Once you have finished all your work on this audit, you should feel very proud of yourself – especially when changes have been implemented as a result of your work.

It is now very important to repeat your work in a specified period of time; this is the concept of re-audit. This is done so that you can see what impact your audit has had and what changes have been made. It is very easy to spend a lot of time collecting the data but the important thing about audit is implementing change.

Re-audit allows you to recognise the effect of the changes which were made as a result of your audit. This will demonstrate to others that the concept of audit really works. It also allows you to recognise which changes have not been made so that you can rectify them.

Remember that re-audit is the last step in the audit cycle: the cycle is not complete without it. It is crucial that you complete the cycle and tie up any loose ends. A common interview question is 'How many audit cycles have you completed?' This often leaves junior staff kicking themselves! It is better to perform a small, simple and effective audit, where it is possible to complete the cycle, than a complicated unfinished one.

The timing of re-audit depends on what you have audited, how big the audit is, the nature of the action plan and your schedule. Often people re-audit in 6–12 months. This allows time for changes to be made but not too much time for you to forget about the audit. Unfortunately, it tells you nothing about the sustainability of the interventions. It can be quite easy initially to get together the enthusiasm to make changes. An audit after a few months will check that the action plan has been implemented. However, sustainability is the real test of a high-quality audit and is the key to effective quality improvement. If you can put into place interventions that last for years, you are well on the way to providing a very high-quality service. Audits are therefore ideally repeated after two to three years. At that time, you will need to review your standards and criteria to ensure that they are still applicable and acceptable to the head of department and other relevant seniors. With luck, you can retain the same standards so as to get an accurate comparison with the previous audits.

In some audits, data are collected regularly to monitor change over time. Although this takes more resources, it can help to show trends in care and to identify when things are going wrong. Following some high-profile cases in the UK, some units are now monitoring individuals' complication rates, to identify those who need further support or training.[15] Although this monitoring caused some initial concern among the staff, it has now been well accepted in the places where it has been introduced and provides very useful feedback for the doctors.

Tips for implementing change

- Changing practice takes longer than you think.
- Create a solid communication structure and make sure that everyone is clear about his or her roles and responsibilities.
- Be prepared to change your plans as you understand the problem more clearly and more people become involved.
- Use the whole process to educate fellow staff to develop problem solving and management skills.
- Be prepared to take risks. Do not get scared.
- The bigger the problem, the easier it is to demonstrate improvement.

Key points for implementing change

1. Do a root cause analysis using the 'five whys' approach.

2. Select appropriate interventions:

   - Is the proposed solution feasible?
   - Does the proposed solution actually solve the problems?
   - Does the proposed solution provide the best result for the least resource?
   - Is the proposed solution acceptable to the patients, community and staff members who will carry out the solution?
   - Is the proposed solution sustainable?

3. Make an action plan.

4. Carry out the action plan.

5. Re-audit.

Exercises

Exercise 9: Implementing change

1. What are the five principal explanations for failing to reach the proposed standards? Can you think of others?

2. Discuss root cause analysis:
    a. What is it?
    b. How do you do it?
    c. Why do you do it?
    d. How important is this step?

3. When selecting interventions to implement change from audits, what five questions must you consider?

4. Discuss action plans:
    a. What is it?
    b. Why do you do it?
    c. What are the advantages of using it?
    d. What are the disadvantages of using it?

Exercise 10: Root cause analysis

1. Consider the first audit problem in your unit from Exercise 4:
    a. Perform a root cause analysis or 'why, why' diagram to assess the causes of the problem.
    b. Select interventions to solve the problems.
    c. Describe why you have chosen these interventions.
    d. Draft an action plan for carrying out the above interventions.

2. Consider the second audit problem in your unit from Exercise 4:
    a. Perform a root cause analysis or 'five whys' diagram into the causes of the problem.
    b. Select interventions to solve the problems.
    c. Describe why you have chosen these interventions.
    d. Draft an action plan for carrying out the above interventions.

Conclusion – let's do audit!

Through reading this book and carrying out the questions at the end of each chapter, we hope that you will have gained an understanding of some of the theory of audit. However, the real learning will only come with doing. So, now is the time to get out there and perform an audit of your own. Talk to your boss, find a problem that affects your unit and get stuck in.

You can use this book to help guide your audit and you will also pick up tricks of your own along the way. But above all, work in a team and enjoy the process. Audit is a process that will rarely succeed if you try to do it alone or impose it on others. So you will need to take your colleagues with you on the audit journey – and the best way to do this is to be enthusiastic and to work as a team.

You will be able to use audit throughout your career to improve health care for your patients. But the time to start is now – so go for it!

Let's do audit!

References

1. Wagaarachchi PT, Graham WJ, Penney GC, McCaw-Binns A, Yeboah Antwi K, Hall MH. Holding up a mirror: changing obstetric practice through criterion-based clinical audit in developing countries. *Int J Gynecol Obstet* 2001;74:119–30.
2. Weeks AD, Alia G, Ononge S, Mutungi A, Otolorin EO, Mirembe FM. Introducing criteria based audit into Ugandan maternity units. *BMJ* 2003;327:1329–31.
3. National Institute for Clinical Excellence. *Principles for Best Practice in Clinical Audit.* Abingdon: Radcliffe Medical Press; 2002.
4. The triennial *Confidential Enquiries into Maternal Deaths* reports, subsequently entitled *Why Mothers Die* and now *Saving Mothers' Lives*; produced by the Centre for Maternal and Child Enquiries (www.cemace.org.uk)
5. Jamtvedt G, Young JM, Kristoffersen DT, O'Brien MA, Oxman AD. Audit and feedback: effects on professional practice and health care outcomes. *Cochrane Database Syst Rev* 2006;(2):CD000259.
6. Althabe F, Buekens P, Bergel E, Belizán JM, Campbell MK, Moss N, *et al.* A behavioral intervention to improve obstetrical care. *N Engl J Med* 2008;358:1929–40.
7. Weeks AD, Alia G, Ononge S, Otolorin EO, Mirembe FM. A criteria-based audit of the management of severe pre-eclampsia in Kampala, Uganda. *Int J Gynecol Obstet* 2005;91:292–7; discussion 283–4.
8. Mbaruku G, Bergström S. Reducing maternal mortality in Kigoma, Tanzania. *Health Policy Plan* 1995;10:71–8.
9. Bugalho A, Bergström S. Value of perinatal audit in obstetric care in the developing world: a ten-year experience of the Maputo model. *Gynecol Obstet Invest* 1993;36:239–43.
10. Graham W, Wagaarachchi P, Penney G, McCaw-Binns A, Antwi KY, Hall MH. Criteria for clinical audit of the quality of hospital-based obstetric care in developing countries. *Bull World Health Organ* 2000;78:614–20.
11. National Patient Safety Agency, National Research Ethics Service. *Defining Research.* Issue 3. London: NPSA; 2008. [www2.warwick.ac.uk/services/rss/services/ethics/statement/framework/hssrec/nhsdefining_research.pdf].
12. Murray C, Kennedy S, Kirtley S. How to find evidence-based advice on the internet. *BJOG* 2009;116 Suppl 1:88–91 [www3.interscience.wiley.com/journal/122589400/abstract?CRETRY=1&SRETRY=0].
13. Mayo C, Harvey G. *The Clinical Audit Handbook.* Kidlington: Baillière Tindall; 1999.
14. Lande RE. *Performance Improvement.* Population Reports Series J, No. 52. Volume 30, no. 2. Baltimore, MD: Johns Hopkins Bloomberg School of Public Health, Population Information Program; 2002 [http://info.k4health.org/pr/j52edsum.shtml].
15. Lane S, Weeks AD, Scholefield H, Alfirevic Z. Monitoring obstetricians' performance with statistical process control charts. *BJOG* 2007;114:614–18.

Appendix.
Worked examples of audits with footnote comments by the book authors

Example 1: An audit of a 'do not resuscitate' policy in an acute trust

S Blayney, A Swan, J Ashworth Jones, M Diwan and D King.
Department of Medicine for the Elderly, Wirral University Teaching Hospital, UK

Introduction

The natural reaction when any doctor or nurse sees a collapsed patient is to resuscitate them using cardiac massage and mouth-to-mouth resuscitation when necessary. However, for patients with terminal conditions this is not always appropriate and may be distressing for everyone concerned. In acute hospitals settings, some patients' case notes may therefore be labelled with 'DNR' or 'do not resuscitate'. This process can be fraught with difficulty: who makes the decision? What happens when the patient's condition changes? How much is discussed with the patient and their relatives? In the UK, national guidelines are available to guide this process. This audit set out to see whether the hospital was following the guidelines appropriately.

This audit was performed in a district general hospital in the north of England. It was started in 2001 and annual data were then collected every few years.

Step 1: Problem identification

Identifying problems

Healthcare staff need to be able to correctly assess the need for a 'DNR' decision to be made and know how to go about this process. Patients and relatives should be included in the decision making, even though this is often a difficult subject to broach.

Is it important?

It is important to identify which patients it would be inappropriate to resuscitate in the event of cardiorespiratory arrest. When this does not happen, patients in the terminal stages of illness are subject to chest compressions and other interventions that may cause needless suffering and an undignified death.

Is further investigation warranted?

Cardiac arrest calls were being put out for patients for whom resuscitation was not appropriate. There was increasing attention given in the media to the issue of DNR decisions and instances when the decision was not discussed with patients and their families, resulting in unnecessary distress.

Is it practical to audit the problem?

Accessing case notes is easy to arrange. It is also possible to interview staff, either face to face or via a questionnaire, to gain an idea of their understanding and experiences.

Can auditing improve the problem?

Gathering data on how decisions are being made and documented and whether staff are being trained effectively will provide a snapshot picture of how well the policy is being implemented. This will inform future training on the policy to ensure it is targeted effectively.

Step 2: Setting standards and establishing criteria

Find the guidelines and other evidence

The Department of Health produced a *Health Service Circular* HSC/028 in 2002, which stated that all hospitals should have a DNR policy, that patients' rights are central to the decision making and that audit of the policy must take place.[1] The British Medical Association, Resuscitation Council (UK) and Royal College of Nursing published joint guidelines in 2007, which emphasise the need for staff to be trained in making this decision and communicating it to patients and families.[2]

Develop valid criteria

A DNR policy has been in place at Wirral University Teaching hospital since 1999.[i] This states that DNR status must be recorded in three ways: written in the current case notes, completed in a specifically designed sticker at the front of the permanent case notes and identified through placement of a blue 'dot' sticker at the front of the case notes. It also states that staff should be trained on the policy.

Step 3: Measuring current practice

Work out what you need to know

A list of criteria could be applied to case notes to determine whether the documentation was correct. A staff questionnaire could ascertain how much staff knew about the policy and what were their experiences around training and implementation.

Next, create the audit pro forma.[ii] This is what we came up with (Box A1).

(i)   Wherever possible existing guidelines should be used to produce audit criteria.

(ii)   By creating a simple audit pro forma, the time spent actually collecting and later analysing the data is significantly reduced. Make sure that you carry out this crucial step.

Box A1.

CASE NOTE AUDIT PRO FORMA

Case note number
Contained CPR sticker in permanent case notes?
One or more sections complete?
'For CPR' or 'DNR'?
Status documented in current care notes?
Blue dot on nursing biographical data chart (where status is 'DNR')?

STAFF QUESTIONNAIRE

Number of staff	
Do you know that the hospital has a DNR policy?	
Have you had any training on the policy?	
Did you know that a patient information leaflet on the DNR policy is available?	
Have you ever discussed DNR status with a patient?	
Do you feel comfortable discussing it?	

Work out how many cases you need

The trust has over 800 beds, so reviewing all case notes within the trust (excluding A&E, obstetrics, paediatrics and dermatology, as these areas do not commonly use DNR orders) on a single day would provide a large number of cases in a 'snapshot' picture.

Work out the best way to find the information

Those conducting the audit went to all wards to examine each set of case notes.[iii] Staff were interviewed from different departments to gain a broad view since the policy applied to all staff members.

(iii) By examining all case notes on relevant wards and questioning staff from a variety of wards, the information gathered is said to be representative of the whole hospital and not biased. Practice could vary significantly between the different departments, so it is important to check them all.

Test your audit pro forma

An initial pilot audit was carried out in 2001 in the Department of Medicine for the Elderly to test the pro forma on a smaller sample.

Collect the data

Use of the pro forma allowed easy analysis of results. The staff questionnaire included free text in some places but the 'yes/no' format for most questions provided straightforward data collection.

Step 4: Analysing the data and comparing practice with agreed criteria

Gather and organise the data

Total numbers were counted and entered into a table (Table A1).

Work out some simple calculations

These numbers were converted into percentages to allow comparison between years (Table A2).

Compare the results to the audit standards

Documentation should be happening in every case, so the score should be 100% for each criterion. Staff training was harder to set a standard for, owing to a frequently changing staff population and the fact that training was not compulsory.[iv]

(iv)   Ideally numerical standards should be set before data collection begins, however this was not done in this audit.

Table A1. The organised data

	2001	2003	2005	2008
Number of case notes	632	574	752	493
Contained CPR sticker in permanent case notes	632	574	752	493
One or more sections complete	303	315	293	281
'For CPR' or 'DNR'?	95	149	135	232
Status documented in current care notes	69	52	684	414
Blue dot on nursing biographical data chart (where status is 'DNR')	51	75	90	89
STAFF QUESTIONNAIRE				
Number of staff	180	201	141	141
Do you know that the hospital has a DNR policy?	176	197	120	114
Have you had any training on the policy?		135	85	96
Did you know that a patient information leaflet on the DNR policy is available?			121	75
Have you discussed DNR status with a patient?	49	92		70
Do you feel comfortable discussing it?	41	111		120

(For explanation of gaps in table, see text)

Step 5: Root cause analysis

Root cause analysis revealed the following underlying problems:

- Patients who were 'for CPR' did not have stickers in their case notes, which resulted in low rates of achievement when auditing correctly completed stickers.

- Blue dots were used for other purposes on some wards, for example to denote to which nursing team a patient belonged. They were also placed in a variety of different places.

- Conversations with patients may not always be appropriate (for example, if it would cause undue distress to a patient already in the terminal stages of an illness). It is also likely that conversations were

Table A2. The data organised to allow comparison between years

	2001 (%)	2003 (%)	2005 (%)	2008 (%)
Contained CPR sticker in permanent case notes	100	100	100	100
One or more sections complete	48	55	39	57
'For CPR' or 'DNR'?	15	26	18	47
Status documented in current care notes	11	9	91	84
Blue dot on nursing biographical data chart (where status is 'DNR')	8	13	12	18

STAFF QUESTIONNAIRE

	2001 (%)	2003 (%)	2005 (%)	2008 (%)
Do you know that the hospital has a DNR policy?	98	98	85	81
Have you had any training on the policy?		67	60	68
Did you know that a patient information leaflet on the DNR policy is available?			86	38
Have you discussed DNR status with a patient?	27	46		50
Do you feel comfortable discussing it?	23	55		85

taking place in accordance with the policy but were not being documented separately.[v]

■ Staff training was not compulsory and relied on 'DNR link trainers' on wards and in other clinical areas to cascade training to colleagues. This was only established in 2001 after the first audit. In addition, a frequently changing population of doctors in training jobs meant that there was a need for regular sessions to capture each cohort.

Step 6: Implement change

The pro forma and the questionnaire were modified in minor ways over consequent years to reflect outcomes of discussions at trust audit meetings and good practice sessions.

(v)   Audit can only say something has been done if it is documented as such. Often, things are done but not documented; if it is not documented – it is not done. Documentation therefore often improves as a result of the audit process.

It was agreed that sticker completion was only necessary if the patients were for 'DNR' and, in future, an uncompleted sticker in a patient 'for CPR' would not be classed as a fail when audited.

DNR link trainers were introduced after the initial audit in 2001. From 2004, there has been inclusion of a session on DNR policy during induction of medical staff and patient information leaflets were also introduced during this year.

Step 7: Re-audit

The full audit cycle can be seen in the results tables (Tables A1 and A2). The most recent change implemented in 2009 is the incorporation of DNR policy training into mandatory basic life support training, which all staff members receive on a regular basis. The audit cycle will continue into the future to assess if this increases compliance with the policy.

Discussion

This audit is typical of many performed in routine practice. Whenever a new guideline has been introduced, an audit can be used to assess whether it is being implemented effectively and whether more steps need to be taken to improve implementation of the guideline. There is no point in having guidelines unless they are implemented. It is crucial to keep checking the audit regularly (perhaps annually) to ensure that staff are still aware of the guideline and implementing it, even after the initial drive of awareness raising.

References

1.   Department of Health. *Resuscitation Policy*. Health Service Circular 2000/028. London: DH; 2000 [www.dh.gov.uk/en/Publicationsandstatistics/Lettersandcirculars/ Healthservicecirculars/DH_4004244].
2.   British Medical Association, Resuscitation Council (UK), Royal College of Nursing. *Decisions Relating to Cardiopulmonary Resuscitation*. London: BMA; 2007 [www.bma.org.uk/ethics/cardiopulmonary_resuscitation/CPRDecisions07.jsp].

Example 2: An audit of postoperative caesarean section wound infection

K Lightly, *Y Nsubuga*, and colleagues.
Department of Obstetrics and Gynaecology, Mulago Hospital, Kampala, Uganda

Introduction

This audit was carried out on the postnatal and gynaecological wards of the large obstetrics and gynaecology department of Mulago National Referral Hospital, Kampala, Uganda, during 2008.

Step 1: Problem identification

Identifying problems

The problem of postoperative caesarean section wound infection was discussed in the daily morning handover meeting several times and comments were made by staff that 'something has to be done'.

Is it important?

This was a very common problem associated with high rates of morbidity and mortality.

Is further investigation warranted?

Yes. There were many questions: Why is it so common? Which organisms cause it? How common is it?

Is it practical to audit the problem?

As it was so common it would be easy to find enough cases quickly.

Can auditing improve the problem?

Postoperative infection was known to be a preventable problem, so an audit could identify specific areas for improvement.

Step 2: Setting standards and establishing criteria for good quality care

Find the guidelines and evidence

It was decided to focus on the management of infection rather than prevention initially,[vi] and both Ugandan national[1] and World Health Organization (WHO) guidelines[2] for management were found. The following advice for management was taken from them:

Definition of puerperal sepsis: 'Infection of genital tract from birth to 42 days postpartum'.

- ■ Swab any pus and take blood cultures in severe cases.
- ■ Give broad-spectrum antibiotics, together with intravenous hydrocortisone for severe cases.
- ■ Use wound irrigation and surgical debridement if necessary.

Develop valid criteria

The national and WHO guidelines were reviewed and a list of criteria drawn up. These criteria were then discussed with the whole team, including junior staff, to come to an agreement. It was also important that the head of labour ward, the head of midwifery and a microbiologist were part of this process. To achieve this, separate meetings were arranged with those absent from the initial meeting. After all, we did not want them looking at the results after the audit was finished and saying that they did not agree with the criteria. Following this process, the final list was:

- ■ 70% of patients with wound infections should have pus swabs taken.[vii]
- ■ 100% of patients should have broad-spectrum antibiotics prescribed.[viii]
- ■ 100% of antibiotic administration should be documented correctly.[ix]

(vi)   It would have been a good alternative to work on an audit of infection prevention initially. However, as the extent of the infection was not known and there were no guidelines for infection prevention, it was thought that an audit of management would be tackled first. A second audit into prevention could always be conducted later.

(vii) Blood culture bottles can be difficult to obtain and so the need to take blood cultures was not included, despite being in the guidelines. Remember, the standards need to be achievable in your setting: there is no point in asking for the impossible.

(viii) Hydrocortisone was only given in severe septic shock in this hospital, so was also excluded.

(ix)   The documentation was analysed in this way as it was already known that the documentation of drug administration was likely to be poor and it was important to find out exactly which doses were being missed.

Step 3: Measuring current practice

Work out what you need to know

Once the standards were agreed, a list was drawn up of what information was needed. This included basic data about the patient, the audit criteria from above, admission details, history, treatment, investigations and swab results. Although these were not all strictly necessary, we collected these additional data while we had the chance, as we thought it would help us to find the root causes of the problem. For example, we might find out that it was only a certain group of women who were getting infected or that the type of antibiotic that we were routinely using would not treat the type of infection picked up on the swabs.

Next, create the audit pro forma. This is what we came up with (Box A2).

Work out how many cases you need

You can do formal sample size calculations but most people take a 'convenience sample'. We collected the data from all cases on the ward on one day (25 patients) and this was considered to be enough.

Work out the best way to find the information

So that we did not miss any cases, all of the inpatient case files were scanned to see whether the patients had puerperal sepsis and, if they did, the files were reviewed properly and audited. We could have gone on a ward round or discussed it with staff but we thought that some cases might be missed that way.

Test your audit pro forma

The checklist was tested on a few cases and then corrections were made as necessary to facilitate completion of the pro forma. We put the questions in the order that the information was found in the notes, to save time.

Collect the data

All the inpatient case files on the relevant wards were reviewed and relevant cases were audited. If swabs had not been taken, they were sent off to the microbiology laboratory by the audit team for microscopy and culture from as many of the audited patients as possible.

Box A2.	
Name	
IP no.	
Age	
Parity	
Date of admission	
Site of admission	
Current site	
Date of delivery	
Diagnosis	
History	
Mode of delivery	
Indication (if caesarean)	
Surgeon (if caesarean)	
Time first antibiotics prescribed*	
Documented first antibiotics given?*	
Documented any other antibiotics given*	
Antibiotic changes	
Swabs requested/taken*	
Other operations needed	
Length of stay	
Swab results	

*Audit criterion

Step 4: Analysing the data and comparing practice with agreed criteria

Gather and organise the data

All of the data were put into one table. This was done on a computer database. Missing results were chased and added to the table.

Work out some simple calculations

Age range, total, percentages and averages were calculated.

Compare the results to the audit standards and identify performance gaps

The results from the audit were compared to the audit standard to identify where gaps were occurring. The performance gaps are shown in Table A3.

Table A3. Performance gaps in the audit

Criterion	Standard (%)	Actual (%)	Difference (%)
All patients should have pus swabs taken	70	30	−40
All patients should have broad-spectrum antibiotics prescribed	100	80	−20
Antibiotics should be documented when given	100	48	−52

Step 5: Root cause analysis

The results of the audit were discussed as a group, with the head of department and the infection prevention team in the hospital. It was thought that swabs were not taken because staff were unaware of how to access them and how important they were. It was considered that antibiotic prescription and documentation of administration was a long-term problem caused by multifactorial issues, including lack of supplies, patient poverty (patients had to buy their own antibiotics), lack of staff, no formal drug charts, and the huge patient volume. As well as these issues, the majority of the discussion was about prevention of infection rather than treatment, as the cultures and sensitivities of the swabs highlighted significant hospital acquired infection. It was considered that infection prevention must also be addressed in the action plan. The analysis is shown graphically in Figure A1.

Step 6: Implement change

Following the root cause analysis and group discussion, an action plan was drawn up (Table A4).

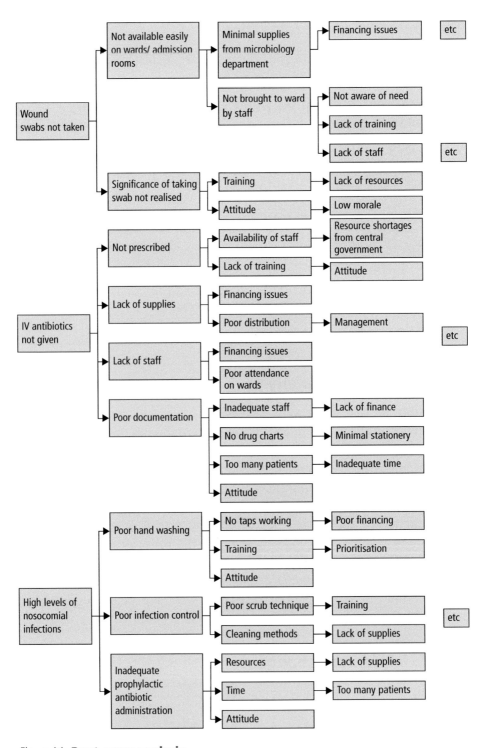

Figure A1. **Root cause analysis**

Table A4. The action plan

Problem and cause	Recommendation	By whom	By when
Inadequate numbers of wound swabs taken for microscopy, culture and sensitivity	Education of importance of taking swabs and high associated morbidity, mortality and length of hospital stay	Dr Lightly, Head of Department	At presentation
	Sisters in charge to ensure swabs easily available	Sister in charge 5AA, 5A and 5B	Immediately
Poor documentation of drug administration	Nurses to put treatment charts at the end of bed	Sisters in charge on wards and all nurses	Immediately
Poor infection control techniques	Teaching of hand washing (the Ayliffe technique) and correct scrub technique; handouts on correct hand washing technique	Dr Lightly	Immediately
	Get the sinks and taps mended by the engineering department and make a new mobile handwashing trolley	Mr Kimuli, Engineering Department	Within 1 month
	Set up meeting between obstetrics and gynaecology department and infection prevention team	Dr Kyambula, Microbiology Department	Within 1 month

Step 7: Re-audit

The audit was repeated in the department three months later,[x] following the same procedures. Improvements were found, although not as significant as hoped (Table A5). Presentation of the findings was used to raise awareness of the issues, and ensure that all action points had been met. Swab use and documentation had improved, taps and sinks were all functional and repeat training on hand washing and scrub technique was completed. A further audit was planned for three months time.

(x) The audit was repeated at this short time interval to ensure that all the recommended changes had been completed. It is not possible to see whether any changes made were sustainable at this point, so the authors planned to repeat the audit again in three months' time.

Table A5. Results of the 3-month follow-up audit

Criterion	Standard (%)	First audit (%)	Re-audit (%)
All patients should have pus swabs taken	70	30	50
All patients should have broad-spectrum antibiotics prescribed	100	80	90
Antibiotics should be documented when given	100	48	63

Discussion

This was a small and straightforward audit which was completed in a relatively short period of time. This meant that the focus of the audit could be the implementation of change. It was already known in the department that there were problems of infection in postoperative caesarean section patients. This audit highlighted those problems, proved and documented them, increased awareness of the problem and highlighted some of the contributory factors, so that remedial action could be taken.

References

1. Ministry of Health, Reproductive Health Division. *Essential Maternal and Neonatal Care Clinical Guidelines for Uganda.* Kampala: Government Printer; 2001.
2. World Health Organization. *Managing Complications in Pregnancy and Childbirth. A Guide for Midwives and Doctors.* Geneva: WHO; 2003 (second edition in preparation).

Example 3: A criterion-based audit to improve a district referral system in Malawi: a pilot study

EJ Kongnyuy, G Mlava and *N Van den Broek.*
Abridged from: *BMC Health Services Research* 2008;8:190.

Introduction

A criterion-based audit was used to assess the district referral system in Malawi. This study was conducted in Silama district, which has one district hospital and 12 health centres. The first audit was performed between April and May 2007. After the implementation of changes, a second audit was conducted three months later, between August and September 2007.

Step 1: Problem identification

Referral between the health centres and the district hospital was identified as a major contributing factor to maternal deaths in Salima district. This pilot study was carried out to improve the referral system by conducting a criterion-based audit.

Step 2: Setting standards and establishing criteria for good-quality care

A meeting by the quality improvement team, comprising of the district health officer (nurse midwife), Safe Motherhood coordinator (nurse midwife), midwives, nurses, clinical officers, anaesthetic officers and laboratory technicians,[xi] established standards for the Salima district referral system.

Standards to be attained in the referral system were agreed as:

1. All referred patients come with a referral form completed by the referring facility.

2. Ambulances are available at all times to transport referred patients.

(xi)   This pilot study involved a quality improvement team which involved senior people in the district and the junior support staff who were going to be directly involved in the implementation of the recommendations. The creation of a team like this not only increases accountability, but also improves team spirit which provides a driving force in the implementation of the activities.

3. Health centre staff inform the district hospital through the shortwave radio when a patient is referred.

4. Health centre staff receive feedback on all patients referred.

5. All patients are adequately resuscitated before referral.[xii]

6. A patient should reach the district hospital within two hours from the time that the ambulance is informed.

7. All the patients referred are attended to by a clinician within 30 minutes of arrival in the district hospital.

Steps 3 and 4: Measuring current practice, analysing the data and comparing practice with agreed criteria

A retrospective review of case files was carried out and compared against the standards. For the initial audit, all of the notes of women who had obstetric emergency complications referred to the district hospital between April and May 2007 were reviewed. For this study, obstetric emergency complications included obstetric haemorrhage, pre-eclampsia/eclampsia, prolonged or obstructed labour, retained placenta, puerperal sepsis, complications following termination of pregnancy and ectopic pregnancy. Sources of the information included the admission register, discharge register, case notes and referral forms.

Step 5: Implement change

Recommendations for improvement were made by the quality improvement team and implemented as a result of the initial audit:[xiii]

1. Two ambulances are stationed in two health centres to serve the other nearby health centres.

(xii) This standard may have been very difficult to measure from the notes, as it is a matter of opinion whether a woman has received 'adequate resuscitation' or not. In contrast, the other standards are all simple to assess.

(xiii) It is unclear how the improvement team explored the problem or developed the recommendations. Although a root cause analysis is not always necessary, it is a useful routine which forces the team to explore all the possible causes of the problem and develop solutions for each one.

2. Healthcare providers (hospital and health centres) have been trained in resuscitation, particularly the management of hypovolaemic shock.

3. Healthcare providers are briefed on the need to handle emergencies urgently.

4. Ambulance drivers are briefed on the need to handle emergencies urgently.

5. All necessary preparations are made to receive and treat the patient when a health centre calls to inform the district hospital about emergency referral.

6. Midwives on duty are allowed to call the clinician and anaesthetic technician directly, thereby by-passing the bureaucracy of first calling the senior midwife in charge of the maternity ward, who would decide whether to call for additional staff.[xiv]

Step 6: Re-audit

Three months later,[xv] the audit was repeated to assess what progress had been made (Table A6). There were significant differences in the demographic data of patients referred during the initial audit and the re-audit. The overall results show statistically significant improvements in four of the seven standards established. The other three standards show a high level of attainment, both in the initial audit and repeat audit.

Discussion

The results of this study show how criterion-based audit can produce significant improvements in the referral system in a low-resource setting. The improvements were seen over a period of three months.

The strategy of the World Health Organization is to reduce maternal mortality by strengthening health systems. Strengthening health systems to

---

(xiv)   The specific action plan was not shown, but this would have included specific details of what actions are needed, by whom and when.

(xv)   The audit team chose to re-audit after 3 months. This allowed the team to assess whether initial change had been achieved, but could not assess sustainability. To check for sustainability the re-audit would need to be done after a minimum of 12 months.

Table A6. Results of the initial and 3-month follow-up audits

Standard	Initial audit (n = 60)		Re-audit (n = 62)		Odds ratio (95% CI)	P value
	(n)	(%)	(n)	(%)		
Patients come with a referral form	58/60	96.7	62/62	100	1.03 (0.61–1.77)	0.848
Ambulances are available at all times	60/60	100	62/62	100	1.00 (0.59–1.70)	1.000
Health centre staff inform the district hospital	60/60	100	62/62	100	1.00 (0.59–1.70)	1.000
Health centre staff receive feedback on all patients referred	1/60	1.7	57/62	91.9	55.16 (10.08–1138.11)	< 0.001
Patients are adequately resuscitated before referral	20/60	33.3	55/62	88.7	2.66 (1.43–5.01)	0.001
A patient should reach the district hospital within 2 hours	23/55	41.8	53/60	88.3	2.11 (1.15–3.92)	0.014
Patients are attended to by a clinician within 30 minutes of arrival	16/52	30.8	50/54	92.6	3.01 (1.53–6.03)	0.001

ensure that skilled attendants are available within a continuum of care has a positive effect not only on maternal and neonatal health but also on a wide range of other services.

This study involved the healthcare providers, senior management and support staff right from step one of the audit. This is in comparison to many other audit projects where the standards are developed by expert committees or universally accepted international guidelines. Involvement of the senior managers at this early stage helped promote the implementation of changes, many of which required resources.

The success of the criterion-based audit in Salima district was attributed to the small size of district, the relatively well-equipped district hospital and the functional ambulance service. However, the referral systems needed some reorganisation to handle emergencies and some refresher training on emergency obstetric care. It is unclear whether the immediate gains from this criterion-based audit were sustainable. As part of the continuing audit cycle, further assessments (re-audit) should be conducted with the addition or elimination of some of the standards.

Example 4: A criterion-based audit of the management of severe pre-eclampsia in Kampala, Uganda

AD Weeks, G Alia, S Ononge, EO Otolorin and *FM Mirembe.*
Abridged from: *International Journal of Gynecology and Obstetrics* 2005;91:292–97.

Introduction

This study was conducted on the high-risk labour ward of a large govern-ment teaching hospital in Kampala and followed a criterion-based audit framework. The first audit was performed between July and October 2001. After the implementation of changes, a second audit was conducted three months later between January and March 2002.[xvi]

Step 1: Problem identification

A meeting of specialists in the department was convened. They agreed that care for women with pre-eclampsia could be improved.

Step 2: Setting standards and establishing criteria for good quality care

Local standards were established using evidence from the national guidelines for Uganda[1] and the World Health Organization manual.[2] This information was supplemented when needed from standard textbooks, the Cochrane database and recent peer-reviewed journals. A set of nine standards for the management of pre-eclampsia was developed, which addressed quality issues related to the management of severe pre-eclampsia. The standards were set to

---

(xvi)   This time frame is probably a bit too short. The interventions will have only just been introduced at the time of the re-audit. It will therefore be fairly easy to show improvements but it will not show whether they are sustainable once the enthusiasm has died down. An ideal time frame is one to two years.

be attainable within the local setting, bearing in mind the limitations of funding and staffing:[xvii]

1. Patients should be seen within one hour of arrival on labour suite.

2. Anti-hypertensive therapy should be started within 20 minutes of diagnosis.

3. Urinalysis should be performed within two hours of arrival.

4. A specialist should review the patient within two hours of diagnosis.

5. Blood pressure (BP) should be monitored every 30–60 minutes when the diastolic BP is ≥110 mmHg.

6. The fetal heart rate should be monitored every 30 minutes when the diastolic BP is ≥110 mmHg.

7. When eclampsia occurs, magnesium sulphate should be administered.

8. A full blood count with renal and liver function tests should be performed in the first 24 hours if delivery is not immediately planned.

9. Steroid therapy should be given in all pre-eclampsia cases where the pregnancy is estimated to be 28–34 weeks of gestation.

Steps 3 and 4: Measuring current practice, analysing the data and comparing practice with agreed criteria

Case files were reviewed and compared against the standards.[xviii] For the initial audit, all the notes of women who had been managed and discharged (alive or dead) from the maternity unit over the study period were reviewed. The notes of women with severe hypertension were selected consecutively

---

(xvii) The very accurate times used in this audit may be difficult to assess from the notes unless there is some kind of strict time keeping in your unit. This could introduce bias and subjectivity into the results. The same is true for the standards of frequency of blood pressure measurement – it may be unclear whether someone who has had hourly BP measurements for three hours but then a gap counts as fulfilling the standard or not. Standards should ideally be very clearly defined so as to remove any confusion.

(xviii) This retrospective data collection is not ideal. First, some notes may be difficult to find. If a woman has died or been transferred to intensive care then her notes may not go back to the usual place. It would be better to keep a prospective list of all those who have severe hypertension so that you can chase their notes at a later stage. Retrospective note analysis also suffers because many of the outcomes that you want may not be recorded. Then you do not know whether the problem is with the quality of care or with the quality of record keeping. Better to have an audit sheet to keep as you go along.

until the sample size was obtained. For this study, severe pre-eclampsia was defined as a woman at 20 weeks of pregnancy or more (or up to 7 days postpartum) with a diastolic blood pressure of 110 mmHg or more, or with eclamptic fits. Proteinuria was not used in the definition, as urinalysis test sticks were often unavailable on the ward. For practical purposes in this setting, therefore, the diagnosis of severe pre-eclampsia is usually made on the basis of the hypertension alone.

Step 5: Implement change

The results of the first audit were presented to members of the department (including nursing and medical staff) at a specially convened unit meeting. Recommendations for improvement were made at the above departmental meeting[xix] and the principal investigator was given a mandate to implement them.[xx] Other changes were also made in the organisation of labour ward by the head of department.[xxi]

The recommendations made by the departmental meeting were:

1. Hypertensive triage should be introduced at the labour ward reception desk. Blood pressures should be taken there and any woman with hypertension prioritised.

2. Two more blood pressure machines should be acquired so that each section of labour ward has a machine permanently available. One should be permanently fixed on the wall in the admission room.

3. Urine dipsticks should be purchased and made available.

4. A protocol for steroid use should be displayed and the appropriate drugs bought. The benefits of this drug should be emphasised in the morning review meetings.

(xix)   No root cause analysis is presented. Although not always necessary, it is a useful routine which forces the team to explore all the possible causes of the problem and develop solutions for each one.

(xx)   It is very important to know who is going to do the interventions and create an action plan. Ideally, an audit committee should be formed to share out the work. If this is not done, it will all end up being done by the person who is setting up the project. This can make the audit unsustainable. It may also make others reluctant to suggest an audit topic if they think that they will have to do all the work.

(xxi)   It is very important to make the whole audit process public and to involve the head of department from the beginning. Without this, you have little hope of succeeding.

5. Because records were often poor, commitment to proper recording of timings should be emphasised.[(xxii)]

6. Charts for recording the blood pressure and fetal heart rate should be drawn by hand on to file paper at the time of admission. New forms should be produced when financial resources allow.

7. Guidelines on the management of severe pre-eclamptic toxaemia should be displayed permanently on the labour ward.

8. It was noticed that there was a gap in care, especially during the morning review meeting. It was decided that the intern doctor on rotation in the labour ward should not attend the meeting but should stay on the labour ward during this time.

Further changes were also initiated by the head of department:

1. A director of labour ward was appointed. The director subsequently reorganised the staffing on the labour ward, giving each member a specific role in the management of emergencies.

2. A fundraising committee was established to raise funds for the drugs and equipment in recommendations 2, 3 and 4 above.

3. The hospital director was lobbied to increase staffing on the labour suite. This resulted in the deployment of two extra midwives.[(xxiii)]

Step 6: Re-audit

Six months later the audit was repeated to assess what progress had been made. For this audit, a further 43 case files were collected prospectively after any woman fitting the criteria was discharged (alive or dead) from labour ward. We calculated that a sample size of 43 would have an 80% power to detect a 30% increase in standard attainment (from 20% to 50%) between the first and second audits with 95% confidence. The 20% figure was derived from the initial audit of 40 admissions to labour ward in which eight cases achieved the standard for specialist review within two hours of admission.

(xxii) This recommendation is quite vague. Ideally, all the interventions should be highly specific and should include an action plan detailing who is going to do what and by when.

(xxiii) The collection of data can be a helpful aid in obtaining more funding. The data were presented to the hospital director, who was persuaded by the results to increase staffing levels. A useful spin-off from the audit!

Results

The two groups studied had similar demographic data and frequency of eclampsia. The overall results show significant improvements in many areas (Table A7). However, no significant improvements were seen in the time between admission and doctor attendance and in the conducting of blood tests.

Table A7. Results of the re-audit

Standard	Initial audit (n = 60)		Re-audit (n = 62)		Odds ratio (95% CI)	P value
	(n)	(%)	(n)	(%)		
Time from admission to Dr attendance (< 1 hour)[a]	13/14	93	26/29	90	0.67 (0.06–7.05)	0.82
Initiating drug treatment (< 20 minutes)[b]	12/40	30	22/38	58	3.21 (1.26–8.16)	0.024
Magnesium sulphate given	4/5	80	5/5	100		1.00
Urinalysis performed	14/43	33	25/40	63	3.45 (1.40–8.52)	0.012
Specialist review[c]	8/41	20	20/42	45	3.75 (1.41–10.01)	0.013
Blood pressure monitored	3/24	12	19/42	45	11.01 (2.94–41.28)	0.0002
Fetal heart rate monitored	0/38	0	11/42	26		0.0021
Blood tests performed	2/20	9	2/22	9	6.67 (0.66–68.85)	0.68
Steroids given	1/7	14	4/4	100		0.03

[a] Median time: initial audit 17 minutes (range 5–2880 minutes), re-audit 20 minutes (range 3–120 minutes)
[b] Median time: initial audit 70 minutes (range 5–150 minutes), re-audit 20 minutes (range 2–180 minutes)
[c] Median time: initial audit 8 hours (range 1–24 hours), re-audit 2 hours (range 0–11 hours)

The number of files in which adequate records were kept also improved. For example, in the first audit of the 'admission to doctor attendance' standard, only 14 of 43 cases had both times recorded (33%). By the second audit, this had doubled to 29 of 43 (67%). Similarly, the number of files containing blood pressure charts increased from 24 of 43 (56%) in the first audit to 42 of 43 (98%) in the second. Of the 258 pieces of information that should have been found in the first audit (excluding standards 3, 8, and 9 as these were subgroups), only 200 (78%) were available. By the time of the second audit, 233 (90%) were available.

Five women (12%) had eclamptic fits in each audit. The standard for the treatment of eclampsia (magnesium sulphate) was given in 100% of cases in the re-audit compared with 80% in the initial audit. In the one case in which the standard was not attained in the first audit, diazepam had been administered to control fits because of a lack of magnesium sulphate.

There were four deaths from pre-eclampsia in the first audit. Two of these were intraoperative cardiac arrests, while one woman died of disseminated intravascular coagulopathy and one of postpartum haemorrhage. During the time of the second audit, no deaths occurred.

Discussion

The results of this study show how criterion-based audit can produce significant improvements in the quality of obstetric care in sub-Saharan Africa. The improvements were seen over a period of six months and occurred in all areas, including speed of treatment, monitoring and drug administration. There was also a reduction in maternal deaths.

There are five constraints to the successful implementation of audit in developing countries. These are:

- the strong hierarchical structure of the medical profession
- the lack of resources to support audit activities
- poor access to scientific evidence
- the poor quality of case notes
- the scale of resource constraints.

We found, however, that these constraints could be overcome. The support of the senior department members was crucial to the project, as was their willingness to subject the department to objective review and assessment. This feature is clearly a prerequisite to any successful audit project. The cost of conducting the audit was minimal, given that scientifically robust guidelines are available free from the World Health Organization and the data collection took time rather than resources. The poor quality of case notes was a feature but this did not restrict the audit process and, indeed, the very process of the audit led to improvements in record keeping. Finally, the scale of the resource constraints is often considered a problem.

Quality improvement may be expensive but this audit shows that a multidisciplinary team within a hospital can produce inexpensive and locally appropriate solutions. Some extra funding was invariably required and in this case the required resources were raised by setting up a departmental fundraising group. In the 'Audit in Maternity Care' programme, criterion-based audit is also being taught in health centres and district hospitals. This audit process has challenged the assumption that all quality improvements need to be externally provided and are expensive. In these settings, many staff have felt liberated to create their own low-cost solutions and conduct their own quality improvements.

The involvement of all grades of staff in the audit process is crucial. While the departmental heads have the financial and managerial power to change labour ward organisation and staffing levels, the involvement of staff at lower levels is also critical for ensuring that the suggested solutions are appropriately implemented. Their early involvement also helps ensure effective implementation and is an important way of enhancing motivation and ownership of the process. This is vital in under-resourced settings where staff morale is often low.

One factor that could have temporarily improved matters during part of the second audit was that a newly qualified specialist was attached to labour ward during her induction period. This led to a marked improvement in the percentage of women who received specialist care and a reduction in median time to specialist review. Although not sustainable, the benefits were evident in this audit and the logistics of having a specialist permanently stationed there is being considered.

Despite the improvements, delays in the initiation of drug treatment remain a problem because of frequent shortages. Attendants often have to buy some of the drugs from pharmacies a distance from the hospital, which leads to delays. Similarly, urinalysis is affected by the irregular supply of urine dipsticks. The huge total budget required for drugs and supplies could not be met in full by the fundraising efforts. A small supply of these drugs were therefore kept in the head of department's office and only used as a back-up in times of acute shortage. To prevent the misappropriation of supplies, secure storage is necessary, even though this can cause delays in their retrieval when they are needed. Our compromise between quick access and security was to have a small quantity of emergency supplies on the emergency trolley, which was checked daily. Staff had to account for supplies used, then the trolley was restocked.

Audit is a useful tool for improving the quality of care. The process itself is cheap and solutions to problems are often inexpensive. It helps to identify priority areas and redirect resources accordingly. It encourages self-analysis and innovation. Improvements may be short-lived after introduction of changes but, in this audit, they were sustained for at least six months. A further audit using the same standards is planned for one year's time.

Reference

1. Ministry of Health, Reproductive Health Division. *Essential Maternal and Neonatal Care Clinical Guidelines for Uganda*. Kampala: Government Printer; 2001.
2. World Health Organization. *Managing Complications in Pregnancy and Childbirth. A Guide for Midwives and Doctors*. Geneva: WHO; 2002.

Glossary of terms

Action plan	A simple table created by the implementation team which clearly records the problems highlighted in an audit and the plans to rectify them. It is a valuable tool for planning, implementing and monitoring activities.
Case notes review	Regular presentation of cases within units for analysis and discussion.
Client	Another word for patient.
Clinical audit	A quality improvement process that seeks to improve patient care and outcomes through systematic review of care against explicit criteria and the implementation of change.
Criteria (plural of criterion)	Systematically developed statements that can be used to assess the appropriateness of specific healthcare decisions, services and outcomes.
Criterion-based audit	The process by which quality of care is assessed objectively against previously agreed explicit criteria. The criteria are developed by a multidisciplinary team using systematic review of literature or evidence-based guidelines.
Critical incident/ adverse event audit	The identification and assessment of cases where an adverse (bad) event or outcome, such as severe morbidity or death, has occurred.
Focus group	A form of qualitative (descriptive) research in which a group of people are brought together to discuss their attitudes towards a product, service or concept.

Guideline	A document with the aim of guiding decisions and criteria regarding diagnosis, management and treatment in specific areas of health care.
Morbidity	The state of being ill or having a disease.
Research	The systematic and rigorous process of enquiry that aims to describe processes and develop explanatory concepts and theories to contribute to a scientific body of knowledge.
Root cause analysis	A problem solving technique used to identify the contributing factors and complexity of a problem and to take an objective look at all the relevant factors.
Service evaluation	Designed to answer the question: 'What standard does this service achieve?'
Stakeholder	A person, group, organisation or system which affects or can be affected by a project or event.
Standard	The level of care to be achieved for any particular set of criteria.
Why? Why? analysis	(also known as the 'five whys' approach) A root cause analysis technique whereby the investigators repeatedly ask 'why?' so as to identify all contributing factors for an issue.

Index

References to the glossary have the suffix 'g'. References to footnotes are in the form 84n.xvii where 84 is the page number and xvii the note number.